Diseases of the Ear, Nose and Throat
Lecture Notes

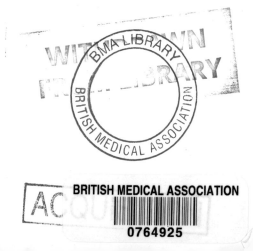

Dedication: For my grandson, Miles.

Diseases of the Ear, Nose and Throat
Lecture Notes

Ray Clarke

Consultant Otolaryngologist
Royal Liverpool Children's Hospital
Alder Hey;
Senior Lecturer and Associate Dean
University of Liverpool
Liverpool, UK

Eleventh Edition

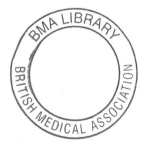
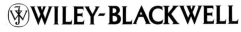
WILEY-BLACKWELL

A John Wiley & Sons, Ltd., Publication

This edition first published 2014 © 2014 by John Wiley & Sons Ltd

Registered office:
John Wiley & Sons, Ltd, The Atrium, Southern Gate, Chichester, West Sussex, PO19 8SQ, UK

Editorial offices:
9600 Garsington Road, Oxford, OX4 2DQ, UK
The Atrium, Southern Gate, Chichester, West Sussex, PO19 8SQ, UK
350 Main Street, Malden, MA 02148-5020, USA
111 River Street, Hoboken, NJ 07030-5774, USA

For details of our global editorial offices, for customer services and for information about how to apply for permission to reuse the copyright material in this book please see our website at www.wiley.com/wiley-blackwell

Library of Congress Cataloging-in-Publication Data
Clarke, Ray (Raymond), author.
  Lecture notes. Diseases of the ear, nose and throat/Ray Clarke. — Eleventh edition.
      p. ; cm.
  Diseases of the ear, nose and throat
  Preceded by: Lectures notes. Diseases of the ear, nose and throat/Peter Bull, Ray Clarke. 10th ed. c2007.
  Includes bibliographical references and index.
  ISBN 978-0-470-65501-6 (paper : alk. paper)
  I. Bull, P. D. Lecture notes. Diseases of the ear, nose, and throat. Preceded by (work): II. Title. III. Title:
Diseases of the ear, nose and throat.
  [DNLM: 1. Otorhinolaryngologic Diseases. WV 140]
  RF46
  617.5′1—dc23
                                        2013024795
A catalogue record for this book is available from the British Library.

Wiley also publishes its books in a variety of electronic formats. Some content that appears in print may not be available in electronic books.

Cover image: Courtesy of David Sugden, Senior Radiographer at the Royal Hallamshire Hospital
Cover design by Grounded Design

Set in 8.5/11pt Utopia Std by Aptara® Inc., New Delhi, India
Printed and bound in Malaysia by Vivar Printing Sdn Bhd

1 2014

Contents

Part 4 ENT emergencies

Preface

'Lecture Notes in ENT' enjoys an important place in the affections of generations of students and teachers of ENT. For many of us, this little book introduced us to a specialty that has fascinated us for our entire careers. For decades it was the standard undergraduate introduction to a subject not always well taught in medical schools, where the curriculum tended to focus disproportionately on the supposed 'mainstream' disciplines. I was conscious throughout the revisions of the need to keep fidelity with what I felt were the strengths of earlier editions – brevity, readability, and a preference for sound advice of real relevance in day-to-day patient care over esoteric discussions, supported throughout by good quality images and illustrations.

The specialty has changed out of all recognition. ENT surgeons are now to the fore in head and neck oncology, thyroid surgery, facial plastic surgery, the medical and surgical management of respiratory allergy and in many of the respiratory conditions that present in early childhood. This has necessitated several new chapters and a radical pruning of some earlier material. To keep the book at a reasonable length I have had to jettison coverage of many conditions that, though interesting in themselves, don't present with any great frequency outside of specialist clinics. I have added a completely new section on 'Emergencies' as many ENT conditions present acutely and good advice on early management can be difficult to come by.

If ENT has evolved, so teaching methods and the medical school curriculum have changed. I have tried to reflect those changes. 'Lecture Notes' may seem an anachronism in an age when undergraduates attend fewer and fewer lectures, but new teaching and learning methods mean that a concise summary of a specialty in a single text is even more relevant. I have included short introductions to the clinical aspects of basic science that underpin the diagnosis and management of common conditions. Students still like pithy revision aids and I have included some 'nuggets' of wisdom in the form of clinical practice points throughout, with an emphasis on making students aware of 'red flag' signs that need early intervention and pointing out common clinical pitfalls. Many ENT disorders still present and are dealt with in primary care, often without recourse to elaborate equipment or complex interventions and I hope this book will prove a useful clinical guide to colleagues 'at the coalface' in General Practice. I have tried to summarize the principles of treatment for common conditions and to identify those where expert help is needed.

ENT is a very clinical specialty with many conditions easily identified by simple examination and observation. Hence I have used multiple clinical photographs, x-rays, scans and diagrams, some of which are from my own clinical practice but many of which kind colleagues and patients let me use, for which I am very grateful. I owe a particular debt to Mr. Peter Bull FRCS, Emeritus ENT Consultant Sheffield, the author of the last five editions of *Lecture Notes*, who was my mentor and trainer and who advised and supported me throughout this revision.

Ray Clarke, BSc, DCH, FRCS, FRCS (ORL)
Consultant Paediatric Otolaryngologist
Associate Dean and Senior Lecturer, Liverpool University

How to use your textbook

Features contained within your textbook

'Learning outcomes' give a quick introduction to the topics covered in a chapter.

> ### Divisions of the ear
> ✓ The ear is usually described as comprising three parts – the **external** (outer), **middle** and **inner** ear (Fig 1.1). The external ear is made up of the pinna and the external ear canal or 'external auditory meatus'.

'Clinical practice points' give insight into how to handle ENT problems in clinical practice.

> ### ⊙ CLINICAL PRACTICE POINTS
> - Suspect complications if the patient with otitis media develops severe headache or neurological signs.
> - Otitis media is still a potentially lethal disease. Intracranial complications can be fatal.

Management and treatment options are shown in green for quick reference.

> #### Treatment of facial palsy due to otitis media
> - If due to acute otitis media, expect a full recovery with antibiotics.
> - If due to chronic suppurative otitis media (CSOM), mastoidectomy is required with clearance of disease from around the facial nerve.
> - Facial palsy in the presence of chronic ear disease is not Bell's palsy and active treatment is needed if the palsy is not to become permanent. *Do not give steroids.*

Photographs, illustrations and tables help explain the topics.

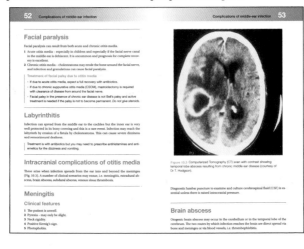

The anytime, anywhere textbook

Your book is also available to purchase as a **Wiley E-Text: Powered by VitalSource** – a digital, interactive version of this book which you own as soon as you download it.

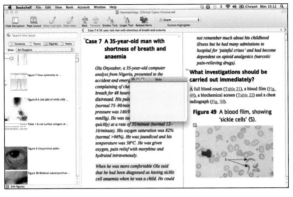

Your **Wiley E-Text: Powered by VitalSource** allows you to:

Search: Save time by finding terms and topics instantly in your book, your notes, even your whole library (once you've downloaded more textbooks)

Note and Highlight: Colour code, highlight and make digital notes right in the text so you can find them quickly and easily

Organize: Keep books, notes and class materials organized in folders inside the application

Share: Exchange notes and highlights with friends, classmates and study groups

Upgrade: Your textbook can be transferred when you need to change or upgrade computers

Link: Link directly from the page of your interactive textbook to all of the material contained on the companion website

The **Wiley E-Text: Powered by VitalSource** version will also allow you to copy and paste any photograph or illustration into assignments, presentations and your own notes.

To access your Wiley E-Text: Powered by VitalSource:

- Visit **www.vitalsource.com/software/bookshelf/downloads** to download the Bookshelf application to your computer, laptop or mobile device.
- Open the Bookshelf application on your computer and register for an account.
- Follow the registration process.

The VitalSource Bookshelf can now be used to view your Wiley E-Text on iOS, Android and Kindle Fire!

- **For iOS:** Visit the app store to download the VitalSource Bookshelf: https://itunes.apple.com/gb/app/vitalsource-bookshelf/id389359495?mt=8
- **For Android:** Visit the Google Play Market to download the VitalSource Bookshelf: http://support.vitalsource.com/kb/android/getting-started
- **For Kindle Fire, Kindle Fire 2 or Kindle Fire HD:** Simply install the VitalSource Bookshelf onto your Fire (see how at http://support.vitalsource.com/kb/Kindle-Fire/app-installation-guide). You can now sign in with the email address and password you used when you created your VitalSource Bookshelf Account.

Full E-Text support for mobile devices is available at: http://support.vitalsource.com/

CourseSmart gives you instant access (via computer or mobile device) to this Wiley-Blackwell e-book and its extra electronic functionality, at 40% off the recommended retail print price. See all the benefits at **www.coursesmart.com/students.**

Instructors … receive your own digital desk copies!

CourseSmart also offers instructors an immediate, efficient, and environmentally-friendly way to review this book for your course.

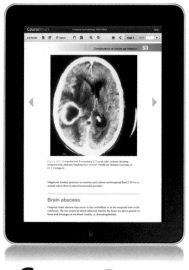

CourseSmart

Learn Smart. Choose Smart.

For more information visit **www.coursesmart.com/instructors**.

With CourseSmart, you can create lecture notes quickly with copy and paste, and share pages and notes with your students. Access your Wiley CourseSmart digital book from your computer or mobile device instantly for evaluation, class preparation, and as a teaching tool in the classroom.

Simply sign in at **http://instructors.coursesmart.com/bookshelf** to download your Bookshelf and get started. To request your desk copy, hit 'Request Online Copy' on your search results or book product page.

We hope you enjoy using your new book. Good luck with your studies!

About the companion website

This book is accompanied by a companion website:

 www.lecturenoteseries.com/ENT

The website contains:
- over 100 interactive MCQs
- key point summaries
- further reading/online resource list

Part 1

The ear, hearing and balance

1

The ear: applied basic science

Divisions of the ear

✓ The ear is usually described as comprising three parts – the **external** (outer), **middle** and **inner** ear (Fig. 1.1). The external ear is made up of the pinna and the external ear canal or 'external auditory meatus'.

The pinna

The pinna (auricle) is composed of cartilage. This is covered with closely adherent perichondrium which gives it its blood supply and with skin. The head and neck in the embryo develops from a number of primitive tissue units known as the pharyngeal arches and the pinna is derived from the fusion of six tubercles of the first of these arches. This is a complex process and anomalies such as fistulas, accessory auricles and deformity of the ear can result from failure of fusion of these tubercles.

The external auditory meatus or ear canal

The external auditory meatus is about 25 mm in length. It has a skeleton of cartilage in its outer third (where it contains hairs and ceruminous or 'wax-producing' glands) and bone in its inner two-thirds. The skin of the inner part is thin, adherent and sensitive. Wax, debris or foreign bodies may easily lodge at the medial end of the meatus.

Diseases of the Ear, Nose and Throat Lecture Notes, Eleventh edition. Ray Clarke. © 2014 John Wiley & Sons Ltd. Published 2014 by John Wiley & Sons, Ltd.

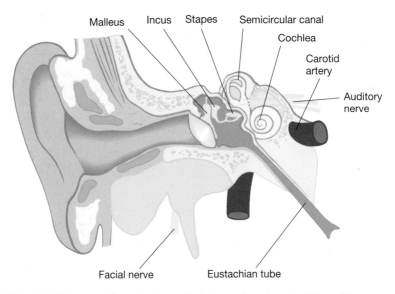

Malleus Incus Stapes Semicircular canal

Cochlea

Carotid artery

Auditory nerve

Facial nerve Eustachian tube

Figure 1.1 Diagram to show the relationship between the external, middle and inner ears.

The tympanic membrane or eardrum (Fig. 1.2)

The tympanic membrane is composed of three layers from out to in – skin, fibrous tissue and mucosa. The normal appearance of the membrane is pearly and opaque. When light reflects off the drum it forms a characteristic triangular 'light reflex' due to its concave shape. If you see this 'light reflex' that is good evidence that the drum is normal.

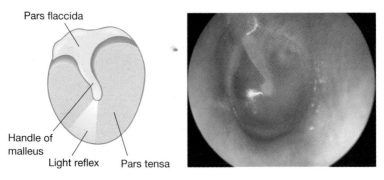

Pars flaccida

Handle of malleus

Light reflex Pars tensa

Figure 1.2 The normal tympanic membrane (left). The shape of the incus is visible through the drum at 2 o'clock. The 'pars flaccida' is the part of the eardrum that covers the upper section of the middle ear. The drum is more 'tense' in the lower section – hence it is called the 'pars tensa'.

The tympanic cavity or middle ear

Medial to the eardrum, the tympanic cavity is an air-containing space 15 mm high and 15 mm antero-posteriorly, although only 2 mm deep in parts. The middle ear contains the small middle-ear bones or ossicles- the malleus, incus and stapes ('hammer', 'anvil' and 'stirrup') (Figs 1.1 and 1.3). Its medial wall is crowded with structures closely related to one another: the facial nerve, the round and oval windows, the lateral semicircular canal and the cochlea.

The Eustachian tube

The Eustachian tube connects the middle ear with the nasopharynx at the back of the nasal cavity. The tube permits aeration of the middle ear and if it is obstructed fluid may accumulate in the middle ear causing deafness. The tube is shorter, wider and more horizontal in the infant than in the adult. Secretions or food may enter the tympanic cavity more easily when the baby is supine particularly during feeding. The tube is normally closed and opens on swallowing because of movement of the muscles of the palate. This movement is impaired in cleft palate children who often develop accumulation of middle-ear fluid (otitis media with effusion).

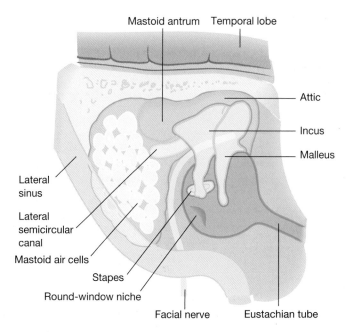

Figure 1.3 Diagram to show the anatomy of the middle ear and mastoid air cells.

The inner ear

The inner ear is made up of the cochlea, responsible for hearing and the semi-circular canals which house the 'balance organs'. The delicate neuroepithelium is well protected in the temporal bone of the skull (Fig. 1.4).

The facial nerve

The facial nerve is the motor nerve to the muscles of facial expression. Intimately associated with the ear, it is embedded in the temporal bone and passes through the middle ear but exits the skull at the stylomastoid foramen just in front of the mastoid process (Fig. 1.3). In infants, the mastoid process is undeveloped and the nerve is very superficial.

The mastoid cells

The mastoid cells form a honeycomb within the temporal bone, acting as a reservoir of air to limit pressure changes within the middle ear. The extent of pneumatization is very variable and is usually reduced in chronic middle ear disease when the mastoid is often said to be 'sclerotic'.

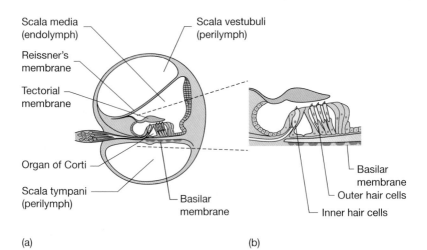

(a)

(b)

Figure 1.4 The inner ear and the mechanism of hearing. Source: Munir and Clarke 2013. *Ear, Nose and Throat at a Glance.* With permission of John Wiley & Sons Ltd.

The mechanism of hearing (Fig. 1.4)

Sound causes the eardrum to vibrate. This energy is transmitted via the ossicles to the oval window which is in contact with the stapes. A 'travelling wave' is set up in the fluids of the inner ear. Specialized neuroepithelial cells ('hair cells') in the cochlea or inner ear convert this energy to nerve impulses which then travel along the auditory pathway to the cortex where they are recognized as sound. Diseases which interfere with transmission of sound across the outer and middle ear cause **conductive** deafness, and diseases in the inner ear which interfere with the conversion of this energy to nerve impulses or with the transmission of these nerve impulses cause **sensorineural** or 'nerve' deafness.

> ### CLINICAL PRACTICE POINTS
>
> - The facial nerve is intimately related to the middle and inner ears. Always check the ear carefully in a patient with facial palsy.
> - The middle ear amplifies sound. The inner ear is essential for hearing. Middle-ear disease may cause some degree of deafness but if the inner ear is not functioning the patient will be completely deaf in that ear.

Go to **www.lecturenoteseries.com/ENT** to test yourself using the interactive MCQs.

2

Clinical examination of the ear

The examination of the ear includes close inspection of the pinna, the external auditory canal and the eardrum. Make sure you gently tilt the pinna forward and look behind the ear. Look for scars from any previous surgery – they may be long healed and are easily missed.

Examine the ear with an auriscope or 'otoscope'. A good otoscope is expensive but a worthwhile investment. There may be an attachment which permits insufflation of air into the ear canal so that the mobility of the drum can be assessed – pneumatic otoscopy. Modern auriscopes have distal illumination via a fibreoptic cone giving a bright, even light. The battery should be in good condition to give a white light.

A common error in examination of the ear is to use too small a speculum; it is a mistake to think this is gentler – use the largest speculum that can be easily inserted (Fig. 2.1). Important points in the examination of the ear are listed in Box 2.1.

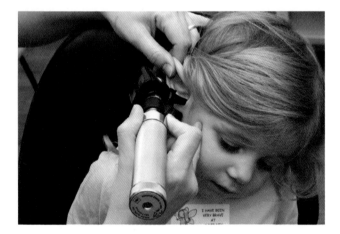

Figure 2.1 The best method for holding the auriscope.

Diseases of the Ear, Nose and Throat Lecture Notes, Eleventh edition. Ray Clarke. © 2014 John Wiley & Sons Ltd. Published 2014 by John Wiley & Sons, Ltd.

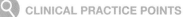 **CLINICAL PRACTICE POINTS**

- Make sure you use the biggest speculum that fits in the ear canal.
- Be gentle; otoscopy in a non-inflamed ear should be completely painless.

Box 2.1 Examination of the ear

1 Look for any scars.

2 Examine the pinna and outer meatus in a good light – you can use the auriscope for this.

3 Remove any wax or debris by syringing, or by instruments if you are practised in this.

4 Pull the pinna gently backwards and upwards (downwards and backwards in infants) to straighten out the meatus.

5 Inspect the external canal.

6 Insert the auriscope *gently* into the meatus and see where you are going by looking *through* the instrument. If you cannot get a good view, it may be that the speculum is the wrong size or the angulation is wrong.

7 Inspect all parts of the tympanic membrane by varying the angle of the speculum.

 Go to **www.lecturenoteseries.com/ENT** to test yourself using the interactive MCQs.

3

Testing the hearing

There are three stages to testing the hearing:

- ✓ Clinical assessment of the degree of deafness
- ✓ Tuning fork tests
- ✓ Audiometry

Clinical assessment of the degree of deafness

When you are talking to the patient, you should be quickly assessing how well they can hear and this assessment continues throughout the interview. Voice and whisper tests are approximations but with practice can be a good guide to the level of hearing.

Make a more formal assessment by asking the patient to repeat words spoken by the examiner at different intensities in each ear in turn. Sit beside the patient and use one hand to occlude the ear canal gently in the non-test ear (**masking**). The best way to do this is to press gently on the tragus and occlude the ear canal. This will mean that the examiner's voice comes from approximately 1 metre from the test ear (Fig. 3.1). Record the result as, for example, whispered voice (WV) at 1 metre in a patient with slight deafness, or conversational voice (CV) at 1 metre in a deafer individual.

If you suspect profound unilateral deafness, the good ear can be more thoroughly masked with a specially designed noise box (Barany noise box) and the deaf ear tested by speaking loudly into it.

Diseases of the Ear, Nose and Throat Lecture Notes, Eleventh edition. Ray Clarke. © 2014 John Wiley & Sons Ltd.
Published 2014 by John Wiley & Sons, Ltd.

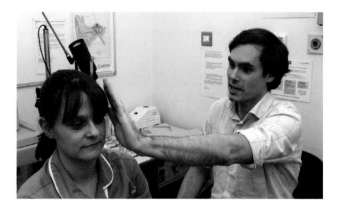

Figure 3.1 Testing the hearing by voice.

Tuning fork tests

Tuning fork tests rely on the basic concept of classification of hearing loss. Deafness may be classified under one of these headings:

- Conductive deafness.
- Sensorineural deafness.
- Mixed conductive and sensorineural deafness.

Conductive deafness (Fig. 3.2)

Conductive deafness results from failure of transmission of sound waves across the outer or middle ear, preventing sound energy from reaching the cochlear fluids. Some forms may be improved by surgery and so it is important to recognize conductive deafness as it is more readily corrected by surgery than sensorineural deafness.

Sensorineural deafness (Fig. 3.2)

Sensorineural deafness results from defective function of the cochlea or of the auditory nerve. This either prevents neural impulses being generated in the cochlea or getting from the inner ear to the auditory cortex of the brain.

Mixed deafness

Mixed deafness is the term used to describe a combination of conductive and sensorineural deafness in the same ear.

Rinne's test

This test compares hearing in one ear by air conduction (AC), and bone conduction (BC). It is usually performed as follows: a tuning fork of 512Hz (cycles per second) is

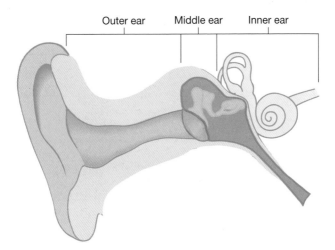

Outer ear   Middle ear   Inner ear

Figure 3.2 Sensorineural deafness is caused by an abnormality of the cochlea or the auditory nerve (inner ear). Conductive deafness is caused by abnormality of the outer or middle ear.

struck and held close to the patient's ear (AC); the base is then placed firmly on the mastoid process behind the ear (BC) and the patient is asked to state whether it is heard better by BC or AC (Fig. 3.3).

Interpretation of Rinne's test

If AC > BC (called Rinne positive) the middle and outer ears are functioning normally.

If BC > AC (called Rinne negative) there is defective function of the outer or middle ear (conductive deafness).

Try this on yourself. Then gently occlude your outer ear by pressing the tragus, giving yourself a mild temporary conductive deafness. Now repeat the test and you should find that Rinne becomes negative, demonstrating the conductive loss.

Rinne's test tells you little or nothing about the cochlea. It is a test of middle-ear function.

Weber's test

This test is useful in determining the type of deafness and in deciding which ear has the better-functioning cochlea. The base of a vibrating tuning fork is held on the middle of the skull and the patient is asked whether the sound is heard centrally or is referred to one or other ear.

In conductive deafness the sound is heard in the deafer ear.

In sensorineural deafness the sound is heard in the better-hearing ear (Figs 3.3–3.5).

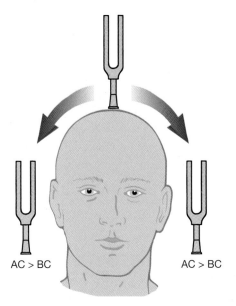

Figure 3.3 Tuning fork tests showing a positive Rinne in each ear and the Weber test referred equally to each ear, indicating symmetrical hearing in both ears with normal middle-ear function.

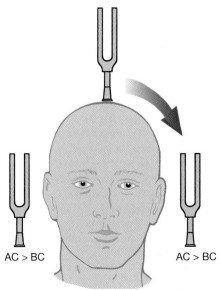

Figure 3.4 Sensorineural deafness in the right ear. The Rinne test is positive on both sides and the Weber test is referred to the left ear.

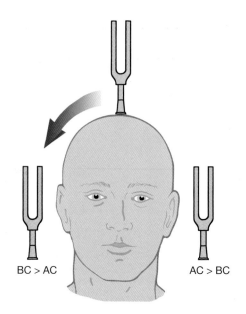

BC > AC   AC > BC

Figure 3.5 Conductive deafness in the right ear. The Rinne test is negative on the right, positive on the left, and the Weber test is referred to the right ear.

Audiometry

Pure tone audiometry

Pure tone audiometry provides a measurement of hearing levels by AC and BC and depends on the co-operation of the subject. The test should be carried out in a soundproofed room. The audiometer is an instrument that generates pure tone signals ranging from 125 to 12 000 Hz (12 kHz) at variable intensities. The signal is presented to the patient through earphones (for AC) or a small vibrator applied to the mastoid process (for BC). Signals of increasing intensity at each frequency are presented to the patient, who indicates when the test tone can be heard. The threshold of hearing at each frequency is charted in the form of an audiogram (Figs 3.6–3.8), with hearing loss expressed in decibels (dB). Decibels are logarithmic units of relative intensity of sound energy. When testing hearing by BC, it is essential to mask the opposite ear with narrow-band noise to avoid cross-transmission of the signal to that ear.

Speech audiometry

Speech audiometry measures the ability of each ear to discriminate the spoken word at different intensities. A recorded word list is supplied to the patient through the

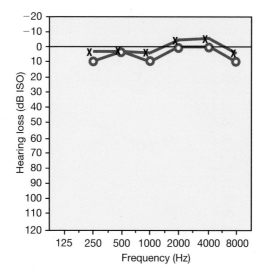

Figure 3.6 A normal pure tone audiogram. o–o–o, right ear; x–x–x, left ear.

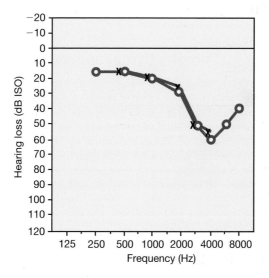

Figure 3.7 A pure tone audiogram showing sensorineural deafness maximal at 4 kHz typical of noise-induced deafness.

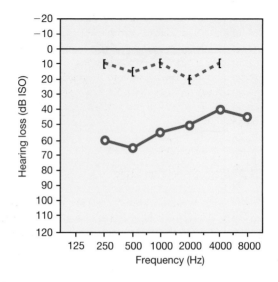

Figure 3.8 A pure tone audiogram showing conductive deafness. The BC (dashed line) is normal but the AC (solid line) is impaired. A case of otosclerosis.

audiometer at increasing loudness levels, and the score is plotted on a graph. In some disorders, the intelligibility of speech may fail above a certain intensity level. Above a critical threshold, sounds are suddenly perceived as having become excessively loud – *loudness recruitment*. This suggests a cochlear disorder and is common in elderly patients with **presbycusis**.

Impedance audiometry (tympanometry)

Impedance audiometry measures not hearing but the compliance or mobility of the middle-ear structures. A pure tone signal of known intensity is fed into the external auditory canal via an ear probe and a microphone in the probe measures reflected sound levels. Thus, the sound admitted to the ear can be measured. Most sound is absorbed when the compliance is maximal, and by altering the pressure in the external canal a measure can be made of the compliance at different pressures. Impedance testing is widely used as a screening method for otitis media with effusion (OME) in children. If there is fluid in the middle ear, the compliance curve is flattened.

Evoked response audiometry

Evoked response audiometry is a collective term for investigations whereby nerve activity in the form of action potentials (APs) at various points within the long and complex auditory pathway can be recorded. The AP is evoked by a sound stimulus applied to the ear and the resulting AP is collected in a computer store. Although each AP is tiny, it occurs at the same time interval after the stimulus (usually a click of *very* short duration) and so a train of stimuli will produce an easily detectable response. By making the computer look at different time windows, responses at various sites in the auditory pathway can be investigate.

Evoked response audiometry has the unique advantage of being an objective measure of hearing requiring no co-operation from the subject. It is of value in assessing hearing thresholds in babies and small children and in cases of dispute such as litigation for industrial deafness.

Otoacoustic emissions

When the ear is subjected to a sound wave it is stimulated to produce itself an emission of sound generated within the cochlea. This can be detected and recorded and has been used as a screening test of hearing in newborn babies. It is now in routine clinical use.

CLINICAL PRACTICE POINT

- Otoacoustic emissions (OAEs) are a quick and non-invasive way to test for hearing in newborn babies.

Go to **www.lecturenoteseries.com/ENT** to test yourself using the interactive MCQs.

4

Deafness

Causes

There is no strict order in the list featured in Table 4.1, because the frequency with which various causes of deafness occur varies from one community to another and from one age group to another. Nevertheless, some indication is given by division into 'more common' and 'less common' groups. Some deterioration in hearing acuity is a normal feature of ageing (**presbycusis**), sometimes associated with tinnitus or 'noises in the ear'. Always try to make a diagnosis of the cause of deafness and start by deciding whether it is conductive or sensorineural.

The deaf child

The commonest cause of deafness in children is fluid in the middle ear due to otitis media. This causes a temporary conductive deafness.

Sensorineural loss is rare (one in a thousand newborns) but nearly always permanent. In most Western countries newborn babies are screened for deafness – 'universal screening' – and delayed diagnosis is becoming less common. Late diagnosis is still all too frequent in poorer countries and doctors and other health care workers need to be alert to the need to refer children early if there are concerns about the child's hearing. Early diagnosis of deafness in babies is essential to avoid irretrievable delay in language development. The mother's assessment is important; if parents or carers are concerned about a child's hearing you need to refer the child for full investigations.

Some babies are particularly 'at risk' of deafness. They include those with:

- prematurity and low birthweight;
- perinatal hypoxia;
- syndromes and chromosomal abnormalities;
- severe jaundice;
- family history of hereditary deafness;
- intrauterine infections such as **T**oxoplasma, **R**ubella, **C**ytomegalovirus Herpes and **HIV** (**TORCH** infections).

Diseases of the Ear, Nose and Throat Lecture Notes, Eleventh edition. Ray Clarke. © 2014 John Wiley & Sons Ltd. Published 2014 by John Wiley & Sons, Ltd.

Table 4.1 Causes of deafness

Conductive	More common	Less common
	Wax, acute otitis media, middle ear effusion, otosclerosis, perforated eardrum.	Middle ear trauma, congenital middle ear pathology, tumours
Sensorineural	Presbycusis (deafness with advancing age); noise-induced; congenital – may be genetic or due to maternal infection such as toxoplasmosis, rubella, cytomegalovirus; neonatal pathologies e.g. jaundice, prematurity, hypoxia; infections in childhood e.g. mumps, meningitis, measles; drugs, e.g. aminoglycosides, quinine, aspirin	Vestibular nerve tumour; head injury; CNS disease, e.g. multiple sclerosis, metastases; metabolic disorders, e.g. diabetes mellitus, hypothyroidism

Children with normal hearing at birth can become deaf in early childhood due to infections such as measles and meningitis.

Presbycusis

Some deterioration in hearing is almost inevitable as patients get older (presbycusis). This starts in early adult life and affects first the high tones. As many as 70% of patients in their seventies could benefit from the use of a hearing aid, and many patients from their forties onward will have marked age-related hearing loss. This is caused mainly by loss of sensitivity of the delicate hair cells in the cochlea. It is usually bilateral but the pattern is very variable.

Otosclerosis

Otosclerosis causes abnormal bone to be formed around the stapes footplate, preventing its normal movement. Conductive deafness results. It is commoner in women, typically presents in early adult life and often progresses during pregnancy. There may be a family history. Apart from conductive deafness, evident on tuning fork tests (Chapter 3), examination is typically normal. Otosclerosis can be treated by surgical removal of the stapes and replacement with a prosthesis (stapedectomy). This is a highly specialized procedure with a risk of complete hearing loss in the operated ear.

Sudden sensorineural deafness

Sudden deafness may be unilateral or bilateral and most cases are regarded as being viral or vascular. Sudden sensorineural deafness is an emergency and should be treated seriously. Bilateral profound deafness, especially if sudden, is a devastating event. Arrange admission to hospital as delay may mean permanent deafness.

Investigation may show no cause and treatment is usually with low-molecular-weight dextran, steroids and inhaled carbon dioxide in an attempt to improve blood flow to the inner ear, although there is no good evidence that these strategies are effective.

Vestibular Schwannoma (acoustic neuroma)

Vestibular Schwannoma is a benign nerve tumour in the internal auditory meatus or cerebello-pontine (CP) angle at the base of the skull. It is usually unilateral, except in the very rare familial neurofibromatosis type 2 (NF2), when it may be bilateral. In its early stages, it causes progressive hearing loss and imbalance. As it enlarges, it may encroach on the trigeminal nerve in the CP angle, causing loss of corneal sensation. In its advanced stage, there is raised intracranial pressure and brain stem displacement. Early diagnosis reduces the morbidity and mortality. Unilateral sensorineural deafness should always be investigated to exclude a neuroma. Audiometry will confirm the hearing loss. MR scanning will identify even small tumours (Fig. 4.1).

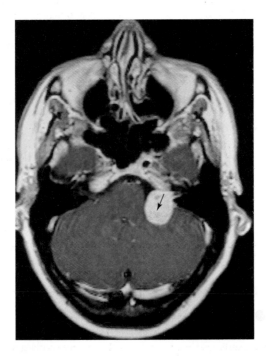

Figure 4.1 An MR scan after gadolinium contrast showing an acoustic neuroma (arrowed).

Hearing aids

Hearing aids work on the principle of amplifying sound. In the typical 'behind the ear' aid a small microphone picks up sound which is then amplified electronically and fed into the ear by an earpiece or mould customized to fit the patient's ear canal. The amplifier is housed behind the ear. More sophisticated (and expensive) are the 'all-in-the-ear' aids, where the electronics are built into a mould made to fit the patient's ear. Some patients prefer these as they are inconspicuous. They give good directional hearing and, because they are individually built, the output can be matched to the patient's deafness. Modern hearing aids are digital, allowing more refinement in the sound processing and more control of the aid. Even with good amplification there can be problems with clarity for many deaf patients. In cochlear forms of sensorineural deafness, loudness recruitment is often marked (see Chapter 3, p.16). This results in an intolerance of noise above a certain threshold, making amplification very difficult. Many modern hearing aids are fitted with a special electronic circuit – a loop inductance system – to make the use of telephones easier (Fig. 4.2).

Bone-anchored hearing aids

Some patients are unable to use a conventional hearing aid because of the shape of the ear canal or due to chronic infection. They may be suitable for a bone-anchored hearing aid (BAHA). A titanium screw is threaded into the temporal bone and allowed to fuse to the bone (osseo-integration). This allows the attachment of a special hearing aid that transmits sound directly by bone conduction to the cochlea (Fig. 4.3).

Cochlear implants

These rely on the implantation of electrodes into the cochlea to stimulate the auditory nerve. The apparatus consists of a microphone, an electronic sound processor and an electrode implanted into the cochlea. Cochlear implantation is only appropriate for bilateral profound deafness. Results can be spectacular, with some patients able to converse easily. Most patients obtain a significant improvement in their ability to communicate (Fig. 4.4).

Lip-reading

Instruction in lip-reading is much more effective while usable hearing persists and should always be offered to those at risk of total or profound deafness.

Sign language

Many deaf children and adults learn to communicate very effectively by sign language. The major types in the UK are British Sign Language (BSL), Sign Supported English (SSE), tactile signing systems (e.g. the deafblind manual alphabet), and Makaton (see http://www.nhs.uk/CarersDirect/guide/communication/Pages/Signlanguage.aspx).

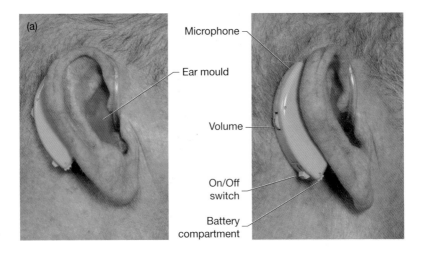

(a)

Microphone

Ear mould

Volume

On/Off switch

Battery compartment

(b)

Naída S SP

Figure 4.2 Modern hearing aids: (a) digital hearing aid 'behind the ear'; (b) a child's digital hearing aid. Source: Munir and Clarke 2013. *Ear, Nose and Throat at a Glance*. With permission of Nazia Munir and Ray Clarke.

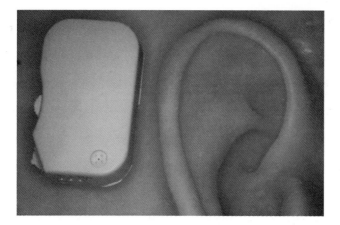

Figure 4.3 A bone-anchored hearing aid.

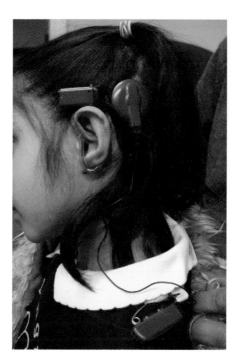

Figure 4.4 A child with cochlear implant. Picture courtesy Mr C.H. Raine, FRCS.

Electronic aids for the deaf

Amplifying telephones, flashing alarms and vibrating alert devices are available to the deaf.

CLINICAL PRACTICE POINTS

- Early identification of childhood deafness makes for a greatly improved outcome. Take the mother's concerns seriously.
- Unilateral sensorineural deafness should be investigated to exclude an intracranial tumour
- In an adult with conductive deafness and a normal eardrum, think of otosclerosis.

Treatment of deafness

- Patients with sudden hearing loss should be admitted for urgent assessment. Although the evidence for treatment is uncertain, they may benefit from high dose steroids.
- Conductive deafness can sometimes be corrected surgically.
- Deaf children need expert treatment. Hearing aids can be fitted soon after birth and cochlear implants have transformed the lives of many of these children.

Go to **www.lecturenoteseries.com/ENT** to test yourself using the interactive MCQs.

5

Conditions of the pinna

Congenital

Protruding ears

Sometimes unkindly known as 'bat ears', the terms protruding or prominent should be used. The underlying deformity is the absence of the anti-helical fold in the auricular cartilage (Figs 5.1 and 5.2). Affected children are often teased mercilessly and surgical correction can be carried out after the age of four. The operation consists of exposing the lateral aspect of the cartilage from behind the pinna and scoring it to produce a rounded fold (Pinnaplasty).

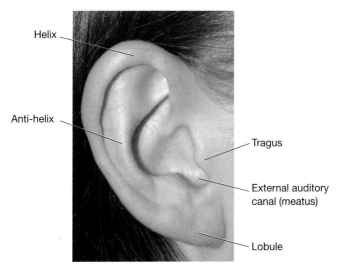

Figure 5.1 Parts of the pinna.

Diseases of the Ear, Nose and Throat Lecture Notes, Eleventh edition. Ray Clarke. © 2014 John Wiley & Sons Ltd. Published 2014 by John Wiley & Sons, Ltd.

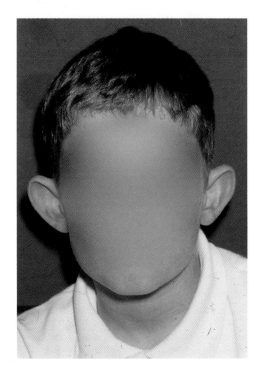

Figure 5.2 A child with protruding ears.

Accessory auricles

Accessory auricles are small tags, often containing cartilage, on a line between the angle of the mouth and the tragus (Fig. 5.3). They may be multiple.

Pre-auricular sinus

Pre-auricular sinus is a small blind pit that occurs most commonly anterior to the root of the helix; it is sometimes bilateral and may be familial. If they become recurrently infected they are best excised (Fig. 5.4).

Microtia

Microtia, or failure of development of the pinna, may be associated with atresia of the ear canal (Fig. 5.3). Absence or severe malformation of the external ear, as in Treacher Collins syndrome (Fig. 5.5), may be remedied by the fitting of prosthetic ears attached by bone-anchored titanium screws (see BAHA, Chapter 4, p. 21). A bone-anchored hearing aid can be fitted at the same time, although it is often fitted at a much earlier age than prosthetic ears in order to allow speech development.

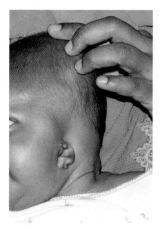

Figure 5.3 A child with microtia.

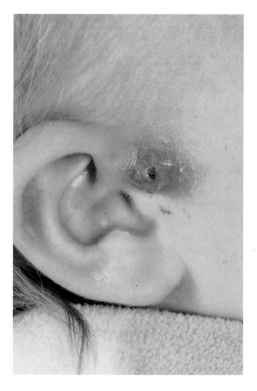

Figure 5.4 Pre-auricular sinus. Courtesy of Mr A Donne.

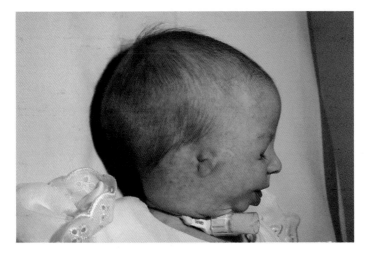

Figure 5.5 A child with Treacher Collins syndrome.

Inflammation

Acute dermatitis

Extension of meatal infection in otitis externa can cause acute dermatitis of the pinna, as can a sensitivity reaction to topically applied antibiotics, especially chloramphenicol or neomycin (Fig. 5.6).

Treatment of otitis externa/dermatitis

1 Clean the ear canal thoroughly (q.v.).
2 If there is any suspicion of a sensitivity reaction, stop topical treatment with antibiotics.
3 The ear may be treated by a glycerine and ichthammol wick, or an emollient ointment.
4 Apply steroid ointment *sparingly*.
5 Severe cases may require admission to hospital.

Perichondritis

Perichondritis may follow injury to the cartilage, mastoid surgery or ear piercing, particularly with the modern trend for multiple perforations that go through the cartilage. **Treatment** must be vigorous, with parenteral antibiotics and incision if necessary. If it is due to piercing the stud should be removed.

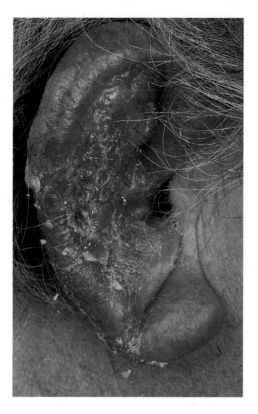

Figure 5.6 Severe otitis externa and perichondritis of the pinna.

Chondrodermatitis chronicis helicis

Chondrodermatitis chronicis helicis occurs in the elderly as a painful ulcerated lesion on the rim of the helix. It resembles a neoplasm and should be removed for histology.

Tumours

Squamous cell and basal cell carcinomas

These skin tumours occur usually on the upper edge of the pinna. They are related to exposure to sunlight and when small are easily treated by local excision. Large tumours of the pinna or outer meatus will require more radical treatment, often with skin flap repair.

CLINICAL PRACTICE POINT

• **If otitis externa gets worse on topical treatment, it is probably due to drug sensitivity. Stop the treatment.**

Go to **www.lecturenoteseries.com/ENT** to test yourself using the interactive MCQs.

6

Conditions of the external auditory meatus

Congenital

Atresia (Greek) is a failure of development; in the case of the ear there may be a shallow blind pit or no opening at all. The pinna may be small (*microtia*) or missing (*anotia*) and the middle or inner ear may be poorly developed or even absent (Fig. 5.3).

Atresia of the ear is a feature of many syndromes in childhood and as congenital anomalies are often multiple, a careful assessment of the baby's general health is essential. It is particularly important to assess the hearing. If the child has hearing impairment, rehabilitation in the form of hearing aids should commence immediately. Correction of the deformity of the external and middle ear can be delayed until the child is old enough to participate in the decision-making. The bone-anchored hearing aid (BAHA, see Chapter 4) and the use of titanium implants to mount a prosthesis have greatly improved the management of these children.

Wax

Wax or cerumen produced by the ceruminous glands in the outer ear migrates laterally along the meatus. Some people produce large amounts of wax but many cases of impacted wax are due to the use of cotton wool buds in a misguided attempt to clean the ears. Ears are 'self-cleaning'!

Impacted wax may cause some deafness or irritation of the meatal skin. It is most easily removed by syringing (see Box 6.1).

Diseases of the Ear, Nose and Throat Lecture Notes, Eleventh edition. Ray Clarke. © 2014 John Wiley & Sons Ltd.
Published 2014 by John Wiley & Sons, Ltd.

Box 6.1 Ear syringing procedure

1 *History*: If you suspect a perforation, do not syringe.

2 *Inspection*: If wax seems very hard, always soften over a period of 1 week by using warm olive oil drops nightly. There are 'quick-acting' ceruminolytic agents on the market. Occasionally, a patient reacts badly to these and develops otitis externa. Do not use them in patients known to suffer from recurrent infections of the ear canal.

3 *Towels*: Protect the patient well with towels and waterproofs.

4 *Lighting*: Use a good light

5 *Solution*: Tap water is satisfactory. Sodium bicarbonate, 4–5 g to 500 mL, or normal saline is ideal.

6 *Solution temperature*: It should ideally be 38 °C.

7 *Tools*: The preferred instrument is an electrically driven water pump with a small handheld nozzle (Fig. 6.1). Metal syringes may do damage.

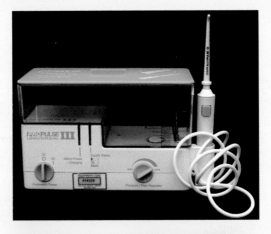

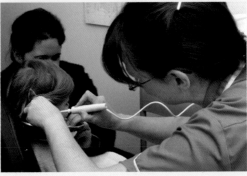

Figure 6.1 An electric pulse pump used for ear syringing.

8 *Direction*: Direct the stream along the roof of the auditory canal (Fig. 6.2).

9 *Inspection*: After removal of wax, inspect thoroughly to make sure none remains.

10 *Drying*: Mop excess solution from the ear. A wet ear predisposes to otitis externa.

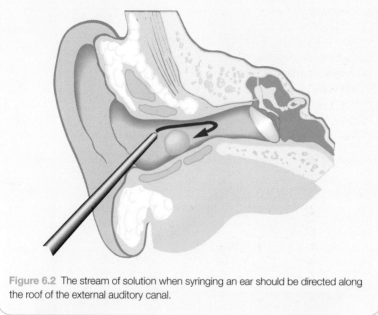

Figure 6.2 The stream of solution when syringing an ear should be directed along the roof of the external auditory canal.

Otitis externa

Otitis externa is a diffuse inflammation of the skin lining the outer ear canal. It may be bacterial or fungal (otomycosis). Irritation, desquamation, scanty discharge and a tendency to relapse are common. The treatment is simple, but success is absolutely dependent upon patience, care and meticulous attention to detail (see Chapter 5).

Causes

Some people are particularly prone to otitis externa, often because of a narrow or tortuous external canal. Most people can allow water into their ears with impunity; in others otitis externa is the inevitable result. Increased sweating and bathing in hot climates are predisposing factors. Swimming pools are a common source of otitis externa. Poking the ear with a finger or towel further traumatizes the skin and introduces new organisms. Further irritation leads to further interference with the ear, so causing more trauma. A vicious circle is set up.

Underlying skin disease such as eczema or psoriasis in the ear canal may produce very refractory otitis externa.

Ear syringing, especially if it causes trauma, may cause otitis externa.

Pathology

A mixed infection of varying organisms is typical; the most common are:

- *Staphylococcus pyogenes*
- *Pseudomonas pyocyanea*
- diphtheroids
- *Proteus vulgaris*
- *Escherichia coli*
- *Streptococcus faecalis*
- *Aspergillus niger* (Fig. 6.3)
- *Candida albicans.*

Symptoms

- Irritation (itchiness)
- Discharge (scanty)
- Pain (increased by jaw movement)
- Deafness (mild)

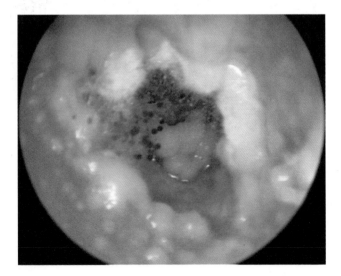

Figure 6.3 Fungal otitis externa showing the spores of *Aspergillus niger* (courtesy of M.P.J. Yardley).

Signs

- Meatal tenderness, especially on movement of the pinna or compression of the tragus
- Moist debris, often smelly and keratotic
- Red desquamated skin and oedema of the meatal walls

Management

Aural toilet

Scrupulous aural toilet is the key to successful treatment of otitis externa. Clean the debris and keep the ear clean and dry. No medication will be effective if the ear is full of debris and pus. Aural toilet can be done most conveniently by dry mopping. Apply a piece of fluffed-up cotton wool about the size of a postage stamp to a probe and, under direct vision, clean the ear with a gentle rotatory action. Once the cotton wool is soiled, replace it (Fig. 6.4). Gentle syringing is also permissible to clear the debris.

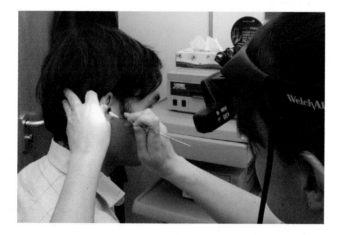

Figure 6.4 Dry mopping the ear in otitis externa.

Dressings

If the otitis externa is severe, gently insert a length of 1cm ribbon gauze, impregnated with medication, into the meatus. Renew daily until the meatus has returned to normal. If it does not do so within 7–10 days, think again!

The following medications are of value on the dressing:

1 8% aluminium acetate;

2 10% ichthammol in glycerine;

3 steroid, e.g. Betnovate (TM);

4 other medication as dictated by the result of culture.

In *fungal otitis externa* you can use dressings of amphotericin, miconazole or nystatin.

If the otitis externa is *less severe* and there is little meatal swelling, it may respond to a combination of antibiotic and steroid eardrops. The antibiotics most commonly used are neomycin, gramicidin and framycetin but there are increasing worries about the use of aminoglycoside drops in the ear as if they reach the inner ear that can cause deafness. Ciprofloxacin drops, as used in eye drops, are preferable. Remember that prolonged use may result in fungal infection or in contact dermatitis.

Prevention of recurrence

The patient should be advised to keep the ears dry, especially when washing the hair or showering. A large piece of cotton wool coated in Vaseline and placed at the entrance to the ear canal is advisable, and if the patient is very keen to swim it is worthwhile investing in custom-made silicone or rubber earplugs. Equally important is the avoidance of scratching and poking the ears. Itching may be controlled with antihistamines given orally, especially at bedtime. If meatal stenosis predisposes to recurrent infection, **meatoplasty** (surgical enlargement of meatus) may be advisable.

Do not make a diagnosis of otitis externa until you have satisfied yourself that the tympanic membrane is intact. If the ear fails to settle, look again and again to make sure that you are not dealing with a case of otitis media with a discharging perforation.

Furunculosis

Furunculosis ('boil') of the external canal results from infection of a hair follicle in the lateral part of the meatus. The organism is usually *Staphylococcus*.

Symptoms
Pain

Pain is severe and exceptionally the patient may need opioids. The pain is made much worse by movement of the pinna or pressure on the tragus.

Deafness

Deafness is usually slight and due to meatal occlusion by the furuncle.

Signs

There is often no visible lesion but the introduction of an aural speculum causes intense pain. If the furuncle is larger, it will be seen as a red swelling in the outer meatus and there may be more than one furuncle present. At a more advanced stage, the furuncle will be seen to be pointing or may present as a fluctuant abscess.

Treatment

The insertion of a wick soaked in 10% ichthammol in glycerine (Glyc & Ic) or a steroid cream is painful at the time but provides rapid relief. Flucloxacillin should be given parenterally for 24 h, followed by oral medication. Severe cases may need incision under a general anaesthetic.

Analgesics – sometimes narcotics – are essential. Recurrent cases are not common – exclude immunodeficiency and take a nasal swab in case the patient is a *Staphylococcus* carrier.

Exostoses

Exostoses (bony overgrowths) or small osteomata of the external auditory meatus are fairly common and usually bilateral. They are much more common in those who swim a lot in cold water, although the reason is not known.

There may be two or three little tumours arising in each bony meatus. They are sessile, hard, smooth, covered with very thin skin and are often exquisitely sensitive when gently probed. Their rate of growth is extremely slow and they may give rise to no symptoms, but if wax or debris accumulates between the tympanic membrane and the exostoses, its removal may tax the patience of the most skilled manipulator. In such cases, surgical removal of the exostoses may be indicated and is carried out with the aid of the operating microscope and drill.

Malignant disease

Malignant disease of the auditory meatus is rare and usually occurs only in the elderly. If confined to the outer meatus, it behaves like skin cancer and can be treated by wide excision and skin grafting. If it spreads to invade the middle ear, facial nerve and temporomandibular joint, it is a relentless and potentially fatal disease. Pain becomes intractable and intolerable and there is a blood-stained discharge from the ear.

Treatment is by radiotherapy, radical surgery or a combination of the two. Treatment is not possible in some cases, and the outlook is poor in the extreme.

CLINICAL PRACTICE POINTS

- Earwax is normal and ears are self-cleaning. They do not need cotton buds, hair clips or pencils.
- Do not make a diagnosis of otitis externa until you have satisfied yourself that the tympanic membrane is intact. If the ear fails to settle, look again and again to make sure that you are not dealing with a case of otitis media with a discharging perforation.
- Meticulous aural toilet is the key to treating otitis externa.

Go to **www.lecturenoteseries.com/ENT** to test yourself using the interactive MCQs.

7

Otitis media

✓ Otitis media is inflammation of the middle ear. The term includes several different disease entities. A good understanding of terms is essential.

Acute otitis media

Acute otitis media (AOM) is a short-lived (usually 1–5 days) infection of the middle ear. If it is viral it may last as little as a day or so but it can persist, causing pus to accumulate under pressure behind the eardrum, which may perforate (Fig. 7.1). Before the eardrum perforates, AOM is intensely painful. It mainly occurs in children.

Recurrent otitis media (ROM) refers to repeated such episodes, typically more than three in a 6-month period.

Otitis media with effusion

Otitis media with effusion (OME) is also common in children. Fluid – often thick sticky 'glue' – accumulates in the middle ear behind an intact drum. Because some fluid in the middle ear is normal for up to several weeks after an episode of AOM, the term OME requires that the fluid be persistent for at least 3 months.

Chronic otitis media

This implies that the eardrum has perforated, the perforation has failed to heal and there is ongoing infection. The term chronic suppurative otitis media (CSOM) is often used to emphasize the tendency for ears with longstanding perforations to become infected and discharge.

Diseases of the Ear, Nose and Throat Lecture Notes, Eleventh edition. Ray Clarke. © 2014 John Wiley & Sons Ltd. Published 2014 by John Wiley & Sons, Ltd.

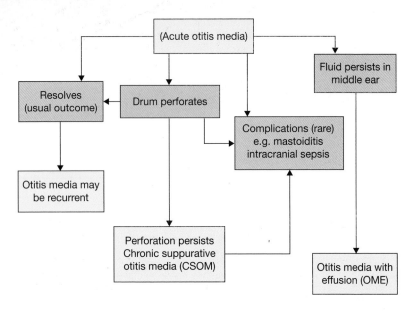

Figure 7.1 Algorithm to show outcomes of AOM.

Cholesteatoma

Cholesteatoma is the accumulation of squamous epithelium in the middle ear, usually in an ear with a longstanding perforation. This is the most serious form of CSOM.

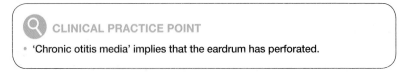

CLINICAL PRACTICE POINT

• 'Chronic otitis media' implies that the eardrum has perforated.

Go to **www.lecturenoteseries.com/ENT** to test yourself using the interactive MCQs.

8

Acute otitis media

✓ Acute otitis media is common and frequently bilateral. Most children will develop one or more episodes typically before they are 2 years old.

✓ It can follow an acute upper respiratory tract infection and may be viral or bacterial. A viral infection is short-lived (1 or 2 days) and often accompanied by some general features of an upper respiratory infection, e.g. pharyngitis and a runny nose.

Symptoms

Earache

Earache (otalgia) may be slight in a mild case, but more usually it is throbbing and severe. The child may cry and scream inconsolably until the ear perforates, the pain is relieved and peace is restored.

Deafness

Deafness is always present in acute otitis media but if the infection is unilateral this can go unnoticed. It is conductive in nature and may be accompanied by tinnitus. In an adult deafness or tinnitus may be the first complaint.

Discharge

Pressure builds up in the middle ear and the drum ruptures. The child gets immediate pain relief but the parents notice a sticky discharge, often purulent. The perforation formed in this way usually heals.

Diseases of the Ear, Nose and Throat Lecture Notes, Eleventh edition. Ray Clarke. © 2014 John Wiley & Sons Ltd.
Published 2014 by John Wiley & Sons, Ltd.

Signs

Pyrexia

The child is flushed and ill. The temperature may be as high as 40 °C.

Tenderness

There is usually some tenderness to pressure on the mastoid bone.

The tympanic membrane

The tympanic membrane varies in appearance according to the stage of the infection (Fig. 8.1). In early infection the drum is red, it becomes tense and bulging and may perforate with discharge of pus. Mucoid (sticky) discharge from an ear must mean that there is a perforation of the tympanic membrane. There are no mucous glands in the external canal. Otoscopy and interpreting the findings can be difficult in a fractious child.

Pathology

Acute otitis media is an infection of the mucous membrane of the whole of the middle-ear cleft – Eustachian tube, tympanic cavity, mastoid air cells.

The bacteria responsible for acute otitis media are: *Streptococcus pneumoniae*, *Haemophilus influenzae*, *Moraxella catarrhalis*. Group A streptococci and *Staphylococcus aureus* may also be responsible.

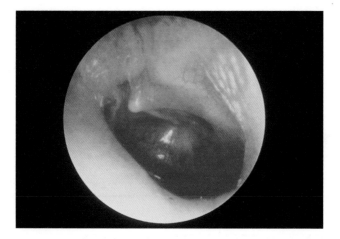

Figure 8.1 The appearance of the drum in acute otitis media.

The sequence of events in acute otitis media is as follows:

1 Organisms invade the mucous membrane causing inflammation, oedema, exudate and later pus.
2 Oedema closes the Eustachian tube, preventing aeration and drainage.
3 Pressure from the pus rises, causing the drum to bulge and perforate.
4 Most cases resolve completely. A small number cause complications (see Chapter 11) or persistent perforation.

Treatment

Analgesics

Adequate analgesia is essential. Otitis media is painful and causes much misery. Simple analgesics, such as paracetamol, should suffice but use adequate doses. Avoid the use of aspirin in children because of the risk of Reye's syndrome.

Antibiotics

Antibiotics are commonly prescribed but critics point out that they should be withheld at least in the early stages as the great majority of cases are self-limiting, and often viral. Widespread antibiotic use promotes the development of bacterial resistance. Some GPs give a prescription which the parents only need to get if the child doesn't improve in a day or so (Safety Net Antibiotic Prescription or 'SNAP'). A mild viral infection can be managed in this way but remember that otitis media is still a serious disease with potentially devastating complications. Make sure you are able to see the child for review and if in any doubt don't hesitate to use antibiotics. Penicillin or cephalosporins such as cefaclor remain the drugs of choice in most cases. There is no need for expensive third and fourth generation cephalosporins in the treatment of uncomplicated otitis media.

Myringotomy

This is the creation of a small perforation in the eardrum – very rarely necessary – when bulging of the tympanic membrane persists, despite *adequate* antibiotic therapy or if there are complications. It should be carried out under general anaesthesia in theatre by an ENT surgeon. The ear may already be discharging when the patient is first seen – *nature's myringotomy*.

Further management

Acute otitis media is not cured until the hearing and the appearance of the membrane have returned to normal. This can take several weeks and a persistent effusion of fluid in the middle ear is especially common in children.

If there is no resolution suspect:

1 the nose, sinuses or nasopharynx; infection may be present;
2 low-grade infection in the mastoid cells.

Recurrent acute otitis media

Some children are susceptible to repeated attacks of acute otitis media. This causes a lot of distress to parents and children but usually resolves as the child gets older. Breast-feeding and avoidance of passive smoking help protect children. Very rarely there may be an underlying immunological deficit that will need to be investigated. If the attacks persist, grommet insertion or long-term treatment with low-dose antibiotics may prevent further attacks.

CLINICAL PRACTICE POINTS

- Eardrops are of no value in acute otitis media with an intact drum.
- Adequate analgesia is essential.
- If antibiotics are withheld, make sure you can review the child after 24 h.
- Passive smoking predisposes children to otitis media.

Go to **www.lecturenoteseries.com/ENT** to test yourself using the interactive MCQs.

9

Chronic otitis media

Following an attack of acute otitis the perforation and discharge may persist – **chronic otitis media**. This leads to mixed infection and further damage to the middle-ear structures, with worsening conductive deafness. The predisposing factors in the development of chronic otitis media are listed in Box 9.1. Suppuration with discharge – chronic suppurative otitis media (CSOM) – can be further classified as in Box 9.2.

Box 9.1 Causes of chronic otitis media

1 Late or inadequate treatment of acute otitis media.
2 Upper airway sepsis.
3 Lowered resistance, e.g. malnutrition, anaemia, immunological impairment.

Box 9.2 Types of CSOM

1 *Mucosal disease* with tympanic membrane perforation (relatively safe).
2 *Bony*:
  a Osteitis.
  b Cholesteatoma – an epithelial sac which erodes the middle ear and adjacent structures including the meninges.

The perforated ear

A perforated eardrum may be asymptomatic. If unilateral, the relatively minor conductive hearing loss causes little or no trouble. The ear may discharge during an upper respiratory infection or if it becomes contaminated by water, e.g. after swimming. Some patients have persistent mucosal infection (active CSOM). In these cases there may be underlying nasal or pharyngeal sepsis that will require attention if the ear is to heal. The ear will discharge, usually copiously, and the discharge is mucoid. The perforation may be large (Fig. 9.1) or very small and difficult

---

Diseases of the Ear, Nose and Throat Lecture Notes, Eleventh edition. Ray Clarke. © 2014 John Wiley & Sons Ltd. Published 2014 by John Wiley & Sons, Ltd.

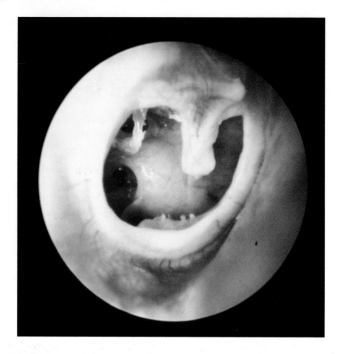

Figure 9.1 A large central perforation of the tympanic membrane. The handle of the malleus and the long process of the incus are visible.

to see. A short course of antibiotic eardrops can help dry up a discharging ear but many proprietary preparations contain aminoglycosides which can cause deafness. Ciprofloxacin is better. Systemic antibiotics are of little use. There is no point in persisting with prolonged courses of topical antibiotics. The mainstay of treatment is thorough and regular aural toilet. A small perforation may heal. Persistent infection can cause erosion of bone (bony CSOM) and eventually infection can spread beyond the ear, e.g. intracranial. Serious complications are very rare but if left untreated the condition may result in permanent deafness or intracranial sepsis. If squamous epithelium collects in the middle ear (cholesteatoma) it can erode adjacent structures and cause serious complications. Surgery is usually needed to manage cholesteatoma.

Myringoplasty

When there is a dry perforation, surgery may be considered but is *not mandatory*. *Myringoplasty* is the repair of a tympanic membrane perforation; various tissues have been used for graft material but that in most common use is autologous temporalis fascia, which is taken from just above the patient's ear. Success rates for this procedure are very high.

'Bony' CSOM or cholesteatoma

The bone affected by this type of CSOM comprises the tympanic ring, the ossicles, the mastoid air cells and the bony walls of the attic and antrum. The perforation is often postero-superior (Fig. 9.2) or in the pars flaccida (Schrapnell's membrane) (Fig. 9.3). The discharge is often scanty but usually persistent, and may be foul smelling.

There are other features of this type of CSOM:

- granulations as a result of osteitis;
- aural polyps formed of granulation tissue, which may fill the meatus;
- cholesteatoma.

Cholesteatoma is formed by squamous epithelium within the middle ear. It results in accumulation of keratotic debris. This will be visible through the perforation as keratin flakes, which are white and smelly. The cholesteatoma expands and damages vital structures, such as dura, the facial nerve and the semicircular canals. *Cholesteatoma is destructive and potentially lethal if untreated.*

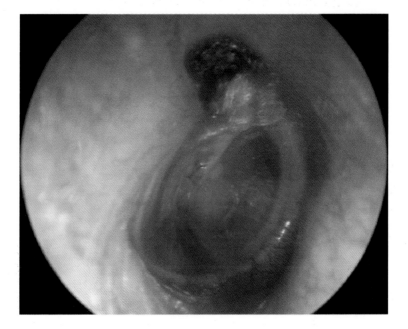

Figure 9.2 Crusting of the pars flaccida suggestive of underlying cholesteatoma. Courtesy of M.P.J. Yardley.

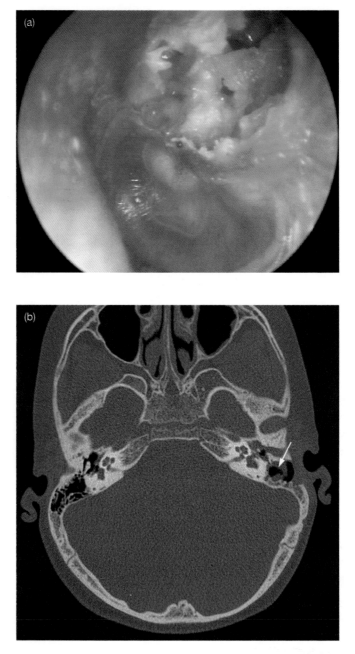

Figure 9.3 (a) Erosion of the attic bone to reveal cholesteatoma. (b) Extensive cholesteatoma in the middle ear and mastoid with some bony erosion (arrowed).

Treatment of bony-type CSOM

- Regular aural toilet in early cases of mild osteitis may be adequate to prevent progression, but such a case should be watched closely.
- Suction toilet under the microscope may evacuate a small pocket of cholesteatoma.
- Mastoidectomy is nearly always necessary in established cholesteatoma. This is a major operation to open the mastoid cells, removing cholesteatoma and diseased tissue in the middle ear and mastoid (Fig. 9.4).

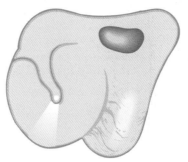

Figure 9.4 Modified radical mastoidectomy; note the shape of the cavity and the bulge caused by the lateral semicircular canal (blue).

Treatment of chronic otitis media

- Dry perforation, with no cholesteatoma can be left alone.
- Discharge can be managed with topical treatment.
- Persistent perforation can be repaired (myringoplasty).
- Cholesteatoma needs surgery.
- Complications (e.g. spread of infection beyond the ear) need urgent treatment.

CLINICAL PRACTICE POINTS

- An uncomplicated perforation may need no treatment.
- The mainstay of treatment is for a discharging ear is thorough and regular aural toilet.
- Cholesteatoma is potentially lethal if untreated.

Go to **www.lecturenoteseries.com/ENT** to test yourself using the interactive MCQs.

10

Complications of middle-ear infection

✓ Complications develop when infection spreads beyond the middle ear (Fig. 10.1). They may be **extracranial** – mastoiditis, deafness and facial palsy – or **intracranial**.

Acute mastoiditis

Acute mastoiditis (Fig. 10.2) is the extension of acute otitis media into the mastoid air cells with suppuration and bone necrosis.

Symptoms

- Pain – persistent and throbbing
- Ear discharge (otorrhoea)
- Increasing deafness

Signs

- Pyrexia.
- Swelling and redness in the postauricular region; the pinna is pushed down and forward.
- Marked tenderness over the mastoid.
- The tympanic membrane is either perforated and the ear discharging, or it is red and bulging.

Treatment

When the diagnosis of acute mastoiditis has been made, do not delay.

- Admit the patient to hospital.
- Commence IV antibiotics immediately. If the organism is not known start with a cephalosporin and metronidazole
- **Surgery:** If there is a subperiosteal abscess or if the response to antibiotics is not rapid and complete, the pus needs to be drained under anaesthesia.

Diseases of the Ear, Nose and Throat Lecture Notes, Eleventh edition. Ray Clarke. © 2014 John Wiley & Sons Ltd.
Published 2014 by John Wiley & Sons, Ltd.

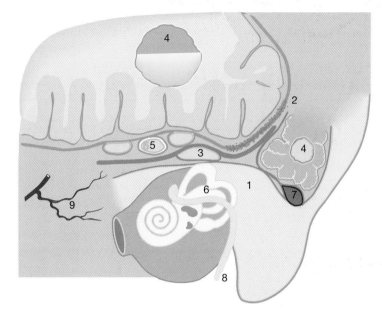

Figure 10.1 Complications of chronic otitis media: 1, acute mastoiditis; 2, meningitis; 3, extradural abscess; 4, brain abscess (temporal lobe and cerebellum); 5, subdural abscess; 6, labyrinthitis; 7, lateral sinus thrombosis; 8, facial nerve paralysis and 9, petrositis.

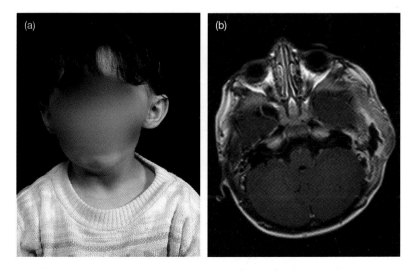

Figure 10.2 (a) Acute mastoiditis; (b) MRI scan showing mastoid abscess.

Facial paralysis

Facial paralysis can result from both acute and chronic otitis media.

1 Acute otitis media – especially in children and especially if the facial nerve canal in the middle ear is dehiscent. It is uncommon and prognosis for complete recovery is excellent.

2 Chronic otitis media – cholesteatoma may erode the bone around the facial nerve, and infection and granulations can cause facial paralysis.

Treatment of facial palsy due to otitis media

- If due to acute otitis media, expect a full recovery with antibiotics.
- If due to chronic suppurative otitis media (CSOM), mastoidectomy is required with clearance of disease from around the facial nerve.
- Facial palsy in the presence of chronic ear disease is not Bell's palsy and active treatment is needed if the palsy is not to become permanent. *Do not give steroids.*

Labyrinthitis

Infection can spread from the middle ear to the cochlea but the inner ear is very well protected in its bony covering and this is a rare event. Infection may reach the labyrinth by erosion of a fistula by cholesteatoma. This can cause severe dizziness and sensorineural deafness.

Treatment is with antibiotics but you may need to prescribe antihistamines and antiemetics for the dizziness and vomiting.

Intracranial complications of otitis media

These arise when infection spreads from the ear into and beyond the meninges (Fig. 10.3). A number of clinical scenarios may ensue, i.e. meningitis, extradural abscess, brain abscess, subdural abscess, venous sinus thrombosis.

Meningitis

Clinical features

1 The patient is unwell.
2 Pyrexia – may only be slight.
3 Neck rigidity.
4 Positive Kernig's sign.
5 Photophobia.

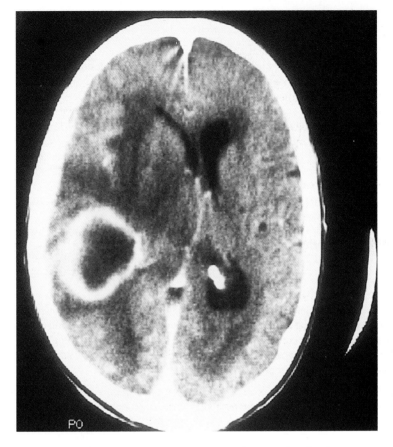

Figure 10.3 Computerized Tomography (CT) scan with contrast showing temporal lobe abscess resulting from chronic middle ear disease (courtesy of Dr T. Hodgson).

Diagnostic lumbar puncture to examine and culture cerebrospinal fluid (CSF) is essential unless there is raised intracranial pressure.

Brain abscess

Otogenic brain abscess may occur in the cerebellum or in the temporal lobe of the cerebrum. The two routes by which infection reaches the brain are direct spread via bone and meninges or via blood vessels, i.e. thrombophlebitis.

A brain abscess may develop with great speed or more gradually over a period of months. The clinical effects are produced by:

1 systemic effects of infection, i.e. malaise, pyrexia;
2 raised intracranial pressure, i.e. headache, drowsiness, confusion, impaired consciousness, papilloedema;
3 focal signs, depending on where the abscess is, e.g. hemiparesis.

Diagnosis of intracranial sepsis

1 Any patient with chronic ear disease who develops headache, neurological signs or any of the features of meningitis – e.g. neck stiffness or photophobia – should be suspected of having intracranial extension.
2 Any patient who has otogenic meningitis, labyrinthitis or lateral sinus thrombosis may have a brain abscess as well.
3 Lumbar puncture may be dangerous owing to pressure coning but is the best way to confirm meningitis. Seek expert advice.
4 Seek neurosurgical advice early if you suspect intracranial suppuration.
5 Confirmation and localization of the abscess will require further investigation.

Computerized tomography (CT) scanning will demonstrate intracranial abscesses reliably. Magnetic resonance (MR) imaging shows soft-tissue lesions with more detail than CT but gives no bone detail. If in doubt what to do, discuss the problem with a radiologist.

Treatment

It is the brain abscess that will kill the patient, and this must take surgical priority. Get the advice of a senior neurosurgeon. Small abscesses can be treated with high-dose antibiotics but often the abscess will need to be drained through a burr hole, or excised via a craniotomy. Then, if the patient's condition permits, mastoidectomy should be performed under the same anaesthetic. After pus has been obtained for culture, aggressive therapy with antibiotics is essential, to be amended as necessary when the sensitivity is known.

Prognosis

The prognosis of brain abscess has improved with the use of antibiotics and modern diagnostic methods but still carries a high mortality; the outlook is better for cerebral abscesses than cerebellar, in which the mortality rate and the frequency of residual complications may be especially high. Left untreated, death from brain abscess occurs from pressure coning, rupture into a ventricle or spreading encephalitis. Patients who recover may be left with hemiparesis or epilepsy.

CLINICAL PRACTICE POINTS

- Suspect complications if the patient with otitis media develops severe headache or neurological signs.
- Otitis media is still a potentially lethal disease. Intracranial complications can be fatal.

Go to **www.lecturenoteseries.com/ENT** to test yourself using the interactive MCQs.

11

Otitis media with effusion

Childhood otitis media with effusion

Following an episode of otitis media many children will be slightly deaf for several weeks. This is due to an accumulation of fluid in the middle ear. Sometimes fluid accumulates without a prior episode of acute otitis media – a middle-ear effusion. Provided this is short-lived and resolves completely it is a normal part of childhood and needs no treatment. If fluid persists in the middle ear with an intact drum, i.e. no perforation, for a continuous period of 3 months or more this is pathological and is termed 'otitis media with effusion' (OME), or 'glue ear'. 'Serous otitis media' and 'secretory otitis media' are older descriptive terms still often used for this condition. Avoid calling this 'chronic' as the term 'chronic otitis media' is best reserved for conditions in which the eardrum has perforated.

Prevalence

Fluid in the middle ear affects most children at one time or another. In up to a third of children it is at some time in their childhood persistent for 3 months or more (OME). OME is commoner in the winter. It is commonest in small children and those of primary school age and may cause significant deafness. It may be responsible for developmental and educational impairment, and if untreated may result in permanent middle-ear changes.

Aetiology

Many cases of OME follow an acute otitis media and are due to persistence of fluid after the acute infection has subsided. In other cases the aetiology is unknown. The adenoids have an important role. Adenoidectomy can be curative in some cases of OME. It is thought that very large adenoids can obstruct the Eustachian tube so that the middle ear is poorly ventilated and fluid accumulates but this must be rare. More

Diseases of the Ear, Nose and Throat Lecture Notes, Eleventh edition. Ray Clarke. © 2014 John Wiley & Sons Ltd. Published 2014 by John Wiley & Sons, Ltd.

likely the adenoids act as a reservoir for clumps of bacteria, which are encased in a polysaccharide matrix and resistant to treatment with antibiotics or to the normal physiological defence mechanisms (a 'Biofilm').

Passive smoking, nasal allergy, and early exposure to pathogens such as occurs in crèches and day-care facilities for groups of young children have all been implicated in OME.

Cleft palate children are especially susceptible to OME. This is due to palatal muscle dysfunction, which affects the Eustachian tube. Children with Down Syndrome and with mucociliary function disorders are also at increased risk.

Presentation and effects

Fluid in the middle ear interferes with transmission of sound so a conductive deafness ensues. This is rarely severe – about 30 decibels is usual – and children can often manage very well. If it is persistent and bilateral it will cause noticeable problems – often enough to affect adversely the child's school performance. Parents complain that the child won't come when called, turns the television up loud, shouts and becomes easily frustrated and bad-tempered. There is no pain, but some parents notice that the child is clumsy and unsteady. Otoscopy will often show the characteristic dull yellowish appearance of fluid behind the drum but findings can be difficult to interpret especially in young children (Fig. 11.1). An audiogram or hearing test confirms the conductive deafness. A 'flat' tympanogram is added evidence (Fig. 11.2). In children under four, pure tone audiometry is difficult and unreliable but an experienced and trained tester will usually be able to get a good estimate of the child's hearing thresholds by other methods, e.g. observing the child's behaviour in response to sound stimuli.

Management of OME

Many children will improve spontaneously. GPs will often try a single course of antibiotics to help shift an established effusion but there is little point in

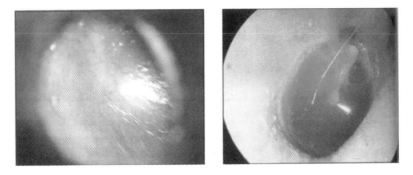

Figure 11.1 OME. Note the yellow discoloration of the tympanic membrane (courtesy of M.P.J. Yardley).

Right

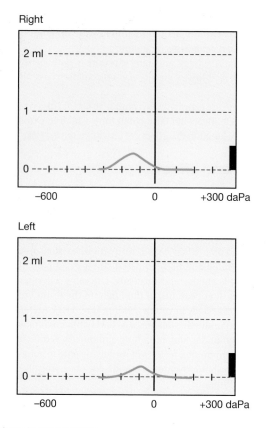

Left

Figure 11.2 Normal tympanograms.

persisting with repeated antibiotics. If there is a predisposing condition, e.g. allergic rhinitis, upper respiratory sepsis or cleft palate – this may need treatment on its own merits. Treatment of OME is mainly geared toward improving the hearing. The traditional approach has been the insertion of a small tube in the eardrum (grommet, Fig. 11.3). This is done under a general anaesthetic following puncture of the drum and aspiration of the fluid (myringotomy). The grommet now permits air entry into the middle ear, which stops re-accumulation of fluid. Hence grommets are sometimes referred to as ventilation tubes or 'vents'. Most 'vents' will extrude after a period of up to 1 year and the child needs no further treatment. Grommets or 'vents' are effective but associated with some morbidity, e.g. the risk of persistent perforation of the drum (about 5%) and of infection and discharge due to what amounts to a perforation of the drum while the grommets are in place.

Adenoidectomy is effective but can be complicated by bleeding. Some ENT surgeons combine grommets with adenoidectomy, especially in children with

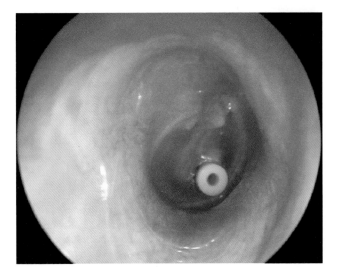

Figure 11.3 Right tympanic membrane with grommet in place.

recurrent effusions or where there is evidence of adenoid hypertrophy, e.g. upper airway obstruction.

Many parents and doctors are concerned about the complications of grommets and prefer to encourage the child to use a hearing aid for a period of several months to a year or so while the middle ear effusions resolve spontaneously. In addition to conventional hearing aids a simple amplification device that the child can wear on a headband (e.g. 'Softband', Fig. 11.4) may suffice in cases where the hearing loss is mild.

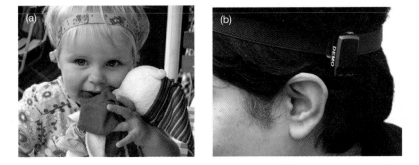

Figure 11.4 (a) Child using 'Softband' amplifier and (b) close-up of 'Softband'.

Treatment of OME in children

- Mild cases: treat expectantly. Advise the parents and teachers re strategies to help the child's hearing. This includes getting her attention before speaking, cutting out background noise and sitting her at the front of the class.
- Prolonged cases may need referral for grommets, a hearing aid, or in recurrent cases adenoidectomy.

Adult OME

OME in adults usually follows an upper respiratory infection. Improvement is gradual and spontaneous, but may take up to 6 weeks. A nasal decongestant – for a short period – may hasten resolution. An effusion can also follow sudden changes in ear pressure – e.g. deep sea diving or rapid descent in an aircraft (barotrauma), can persist after an episode of acute otitis media as in children or may be a sign of Eustachian tube obstruction. Rarely it can be a presentation of nasopharyngeal malignancy. If there is no obvious explanation such as barotrauma or a recent ear infection examination of the nasopharynx to exclude tumour is essential.

> **CLINICAL PRACTICE POINTS**
>
> - Fluid in the middle ear is a normal event in childhood. It only needs treatment if it is persistent and causes deafness.
> - Think of a nasopharyngeal tumour in an adult with an unexplained middle ear effusion.

 Go to **www.lecturenoteseries.com/ENT** to test yourself using the interactive MCQs.

12

Earache (otalgia)

✓ Earache may be due to ear disease (aural causes), or to disease elsewhere (referred earache).

Aural causes

The most common causes are:

- *acute otitis media,*
- *acute otitis externa, furunculosis* and, rarely,
- *acute mastoiditis.*

Malignant disease of the ear may cause intractable earache.

Referred earache

In referred pain pathology in a structure supplied by a sensory nerve can cause pain to be felt in another structure supplied by that same nerve. The ear has a rich nerve supply and is especially susceptible. Figure 12.1 shows the sensory nerve supply of some of the structures of the head and neck and helps to explain why referred earache is so common. Examples of structures that cause earache due to referred pain are:

- teeth, temporomandibular joint or the tongue (trigeminal nerve, auriculo-temporal branch);
- the tonsil and the tongue base (glossopharyngeal nerve); earache can be very severe after tonsillectomy;
- the larynx or pharynx;
- the neck (great auricular and lesser occipital nerves).

Diseases of the Ear, Nose and Throat Lecture Notes, Eleventh edition. Ray Clarke. © 2014 John Wiley & Sons Ltd.
Published 2014 by John Wiley & Sons, Ltd.

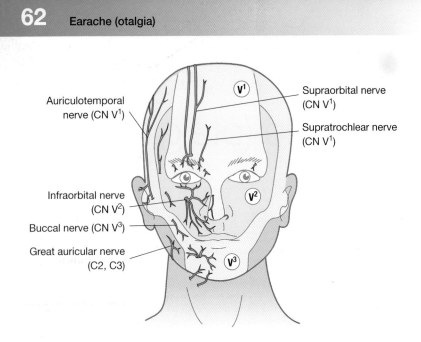

Figure 12.1 Sensory nerve supply of the head and neck. V1, V2 and V3: first, second and third divisions of the trigeminal nerve; CN: cranial nerve; C: cervical nerve.

CLINICAL PRACTICE POINT

- If the ear is normal on examination, look for a source of referred pain.

Go to **www.lecturenoteseries.com/ENT** to test yourself using the interactive MCQs.

13

Tinnitus

Tinnitus is the complaint of noises in the ears in the absence of a sound stimulus. Most patients will report this as ringing, buzzing, crackling or hissing. It is not a disease but a symptom. Most people experience transient tinnitus at some time, particularly after exposure to loud noise. The exact cause is unknown but it is thought to be due to inappropriate activity in the hair cells of the cochlea. There are multiple possible causes but most cases are idiopathic (see Box 15.1). It is especially common in diseases such as presbycusis which affect hair cell function. It can be a very unwelcome feature of advancing age. Most tinnitus patients notice that the noises are worse in quiet surroundings. Tinnitus is aggravated by fatigue, anxiety and depression.

Box 13.1 Local and general causes of tinnitus

Local causes

Tinnitus may be a symptom of any abnormal condition of the ear and may be associated with any form of deafness.

- Presbycusis – often causes tinnitus.
- Menière's disease – tinnitus is usually worse with the acute attacks.
- Noise-induced deafness – tinnitus may be worse immediately after exposure to noise.
- Aneurysm, vascular malformation and some vascular intracranial tumours, e.g. glomus jugulare tumour can cause 'pulsatile' tinnitus, which may even be heard by an examiner. Listen to the side of the head with a stethoscope.

General causes

Tinnitus is often a feature of general ill-health as in:

- fever;
- cardiovascular disease – hypertension, atheroma, cardiac failure;
- blood disease – anaemia, raised viscosity;
- neurological disease – multiple sclerosis, neuropathy;
- drug treatment – aspirin, quinine, ototoxic drugs;
- alcohol abuse.

Diseases of the Ear, Nose and Throat Lecture Notes, Eleventh edition. Ray Clarke. © 2014 John Wiley & Sons Ltd.
Published 2014 by John Wiley & Sons, Ltd.

Management

Management focuses on excluding treatable causes and helping patients cope.
Tinnitus due to chronic degeneration, such as presbycusis, ototoxicity or noise-induced deafness, is usually permanent. With time, the tinnitus will obtrude less as the patient adjusts to it and avoids circumstances that aggravate it. It very rarely goes away completely.

Take the patient's fears and complaints seriously. Take a thorough history and examine the patient properly. Many patients fear that tinnitus indicates serious disease of the ear or a brain tumour. Always test the hearing. If you find an abnormality of the ear such as impacted wax or otitis media, treatment will often cure the tinnitus.

Patients with depression are particularly susceptible to the effects of tinnitus. Severe tinnitus may precipitate depression and patients may need expert help.

Drug treatment, such as sedatives and antidepressants, may help the patient but will not eliminate tinnitus. Anticonvulsant drugs and vasodilators may be of benefit but their effectiveness cannot be predicted.

If the patient with tinnitus is also deaf, a hearing aid is very helpful not only to rehabilitate the hearing loss but in 'masking' the tinnitus.

'Tinnitus maskers' or 'white noise generators' will also make tinnitus less obtrusive. A typical device looks like a post-aural or 'behind the ear' hearing aid and its output characteristics can be adjusted to obtain the most effective frequency and intensity.

If the patient is kept awake by tinnitus, a radio with a time switch may help. Many patients use a 'pillow masker' obtainable in most electrical stores, which emits a constant low intensity sound that helps patients to focus on a sound other than the tinnitus that is often easier to tolerate.

Many patients use relaxation techniques, acupuncture and herbal remedies.

Patients will often read of new 'cures' for tinnitus in the popular press. Sadly these will almost always prove useless and cause more distress and disappointment when it transpires they don't work.

Patients who are very distressed may find counselling by a skilled hearing therapist helpful.

It is helpful for patients to understand that this is an extremely common problem and the British Tinnitus Association website (www.tinnitus.org.uk) can be a useful resource.

Q CLINICAL PRACTICE POINTS

- Tinnitus can be an extremely distressing complaint. Treat it and the patient seriously.
- Most cases are idiopathic.
- Beware supposed new 'cures' for tinnitus.

Go to **www.lecturenoteseries.com/ENT** to test yourself using the interactive MCQs.

14

Balance disorders

Applied physiology

The physiology of balance is complex (Fig. 14.1). The body's sense of equilibrium is maintained by input from a number of sources. These include the eyes, proprioceptive organs especially in the muscles and joints of the neck, peripheral nerves, the labyrinth or 'balance organ' in the inner ear which includes the *vestibule* and *semicircular canals* and the cerebral cortex and cerebellum. Input from all these sources converges in the brain stem; dysfunction of any of these systems may lead to imbalance, a feeling of unsteadiness, 'vertigo' – a sensation of movement – and a tendency to fall. Vertigo may be accompanied by 'nystagmus' – a rapid beating of the eyes to one side as impulses from the brain stem to the ocular muscles attempt to correct the patient's balance. Balance disorders are common, particularly in the elderly. They can be extremely disabling, restricting patients' ability to look after themselves and causing great distress. 'Dizzy' patients often believe they have developed a serious and incurable disease but most cases are due to benign and often self-limiting pathology.

Diagnosis

Some of the main causes are listed in Table 14.1. The diagnosis of the cause of vertigo or imbalance depends mostly on history, much on examination and little on investigation. Patients will use various terms to describe their imbalance including 'dizziness', 'vertigo', 'funny turns' and giddiness'. A careful history is by far the most important aspect of assessing balance disorders. Patients can mean very different things by the terms they use so take time to listen to and understand exactly what sensation the patient is complaining of. Pay particular

Diseases of the Ear, Nose and Throat Lecture Notes, Eleventh edition. Ray Clarke. © 2014 John Wiley & Sons Ltd.
Published 2014 by John Wiley & Sons, Ltd.

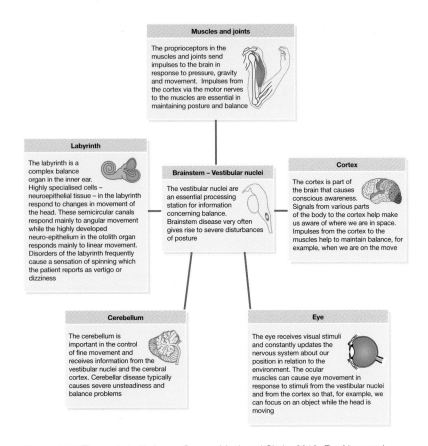

Figure 14.1 The control of balance. Source: Munir and Clarke 2013. *Ear, Nose and Throat at a Glance*. With permission of John Wiley & Sons Ltd.

attention to *timing*, i.e. are the symptoms constant or episodic; are they short-lived as in the few minutes of dizziness associated with benign positional vertigo, or do they last for a few hours as in Menière's disease; are there associated *ear symptoms*, e.g. deafness, tinnitus, earache or discharge; and are there *neurological* features, i.e. loss of consciousness, weakness, numbness, dysarthria and diplopia, or seizures. Note the *past medical history* and make a record of the patient's *medications*. The causes of balance disorders can be multifactorial, especially in the elderly.

Table 14.1 Guide to causes of vertigo

Episodic with ear symptoms
- Migraine
- Menie`re's disease

Episodic without ear symptoms
- Migraine
- Benign paroxysmal positional vertigo
- Transient ischaemic attacks
- Epilepsy
- Cardiac dysrhythmia
- Postural hypotension
- Cervical spondylosis

Constant with ear symptoms
- Chronic otitis media with labyrinthine fistula
- Ototoxicity
- Acoustic neuroma

Constant without aural symptoms
- Multiple sclerosis
- Intracranial tumour
- Cardiovascular disease
- Degenerative disorder of the vestibular labyrinth
- Hyperventilation
- Alcoholism

Solitary acute attack with ear symptoms
- Viral infection, e.g. mumps, herpes zoster
- Vascular occlusion
- Labyrinthine fistula
- Round-window membrane rupture/head injury

Solitary acute attack without aural symptoms
- Acute labyrinthitis
- Vasovagal faint
- Vestibular neuronitis
- Trauma

Common specific disorders

Benign paroxysmal positional vertigo

In benign paroxysmal positional vertigo (BPPV) short-lived (often a few seconds) attacks of vertigo are precipitated by turning the head, especially when the patient is in bed. A sensation that the head is 'spinning' occurs following a latent period of several seconds. This is thought to be due to a degenerative condition of the utricle of the inner ear which causes calcified particles to shear off the highly specialized neuro-epithelium. BPPV may occur spontaneously or following head injury. It is also seen in chronic otitis media. The symptoms can be reproduced by rapidly turning the patient's head while she is lying on an examination couch with her head gently lowered below the head of the couch and supported firmly by the examiner (Hallpike Positional Manoeuvre). Nystagmus will be seen but repeated testing results in abolition of the vertigo. Steady resolution of BPPV is to be expected over a period of weeks or months. It may be recurrent.

Treatment

BPPV can often be relieved completely by the Epley or 'particle repositioning' manoeuvre. This is a series of sequential controlled movements of the head usually carried out by a skilled audiologist which is said to work by dislodging calcified particles ('otoliths') within the inner ear fluids.

Menière's disease

Menière's disease is fortunately uncommon, but may be incapacitating. This is a condition of unknown aetiology but interest has focused on distension of the structures in the inner ear by retained fluid. There is a typical triad of symptoms of vertigo, deafness and tinnitus. The attacks can last from a few hours to several days. Vomiting is common during attacks. It can occur at any age, but its onset is most common between 40 and 60 years. It usually starts in one ear, but the second becomes affected in 25% of cases. Although deafness is fluctuant repeated attacks can cause significant sensorineural hearing loss. Tinnitus may be constant but is more severe before an attack.

Treatment
Medical

Anti-emetics and labyrinthine sedatives are helpful in an acute attack, but if the patient is vomiting oral medication is of limited value. Cinnarizine and prochlorperazine are useful. Prochlorperazine can be given as a suppository or sublabially, or chlorpromazine may be given as an intramuscular injection. Between attacks, various methods of treatment are used but the evidence for their efficacy is weak. They include:

- fluid and salt restriction;
- avoidance of smoking and excessive alcohol or coffee;
- regular therapy with betahistine hydrochloride;
- labyrinthine sedatives, e.g. cinnarizine or prochlorperazine;
- low-dose diuretic therapy.

Surgical

Some ENT surgeons will offer surgery for patients with severe disabling Menière's disease which cannot be controlled by the above measures. Techniques include labyrinthectomy but as this destroys the hearing it is only considered in unilateral cases and when the hearing is already severely impaired. An alternative is the instillation of an ototoxic drug such as gentamycin into the inner ear. There is a significant risk to hearing with this technique. Surgical division of the vestibular nerve preserves the hearing but is a hazardous procedure.

Vertebrobasilar insufficiency

Ischaemia in the part of the brain supplied by the vertebrobasilar artery can cause momentary attacks of vertigo. These are typically precipitated by neck extension, e.g. hanging washing on a line. The diagnosis is more certain if other features of brain stem ischaemia such as dysarthria or diplopia, are present. Severe ischaemia may cause 'drop attacks' without loss of consciousness.

Ototoxic drugs

Ototoxic drugs, such as gentamycin and other aminoglycoside antibiotics, can cause disabling and permanent loss of balance by destruction of labyrinthine function. The risk is reduced by careful monitoring of serum levels of the drug, especially in patients with renal impairment. There is not usually any rotational vertigo, just a sensation of poor balance control (ataxia).

Acute labyrinthitis

Acute suppurative or pyogenic labyrinthitis causes severe vertigo and total loss of hearing. This can complicate otitis media. The term 'acute labyrinthitis' is also used to describe a sudden onset of vertigo of unknown aetiology associated with vomiting and in severe cases collapse. Nystagmus is a prominent feature. The structures in the labyrinth include both the vestibule, which is concerned with balance and the cochlea. If the hearing is unaffected it is assumed that rather than affecting the entire labyrinth the cochlea is spared and the term vestibular neuronitis is used. A viral cause is often assumed. Some cases may be due to a vascular event. To emphasize the uncertainty over aetiology many authors prefer the term 'acute vestibular failure' or 'recurrent vestibulopathy'. Management is similar to that of Menière's disease in the acute phase. Improvement takes place over a period of weeks and is quicker in younger patients. There may be residual imbalance which can take months or years to resolve.

Trauma to the labyrinth

Trauma to the labyrinth causing vertigo may complicate head injury, with or without temporal bone fracture. Vertigo may occur after ear surgery and will usually settle in a few days.

CLINICAL PRACTICE POINT

- Acute loss of balance is extremely frightening. Many patients will suspect they have developed a brain tumour or some serious disease but most of the causes of balance disorders are benign.

Treatment of balance disorders

- Treat the underlying cause if you can, e.g. cardiovascular disease, epilepsy.
- Antihistamines and vestibular 'sedatives' can be used in acute attacks.
- BPV often responds well to 'Epley's Manouvre'.
- Surgery has a very limited role.

Go to **www.lecturenoteseries.com/ENT** to test yourself using the interactive MCQs.

15

Facial nerve paralysis

Applied anatomy and physiology

The facial (seventh cranial, VII) nerve provides motor fibres to the muscles of facial expression. It originates in the seventh nerve nucleus in the brain stem (pons), enters the middle ear and mastoid and exits the skull at the stylomastoid foramen just in front of the mastoid process. From here it enters the parotid gland where it divides into its branches (Fig. 15.1). Paralysis can be caused by pathology anywhere along the nerve course or in the cortical nerves which control the nucleus (supranuclear or upper motor neurone fibres) resulting in asymmetric movement of some or all of the muscles of facial expression. Facial nerve palsy causes difficulty with smiling, frowning and expressing emotions. It is a devastating condition for the patient. The causes are numerous and are considered in Table 15.1.

'Supranuclear' or upper motor neurone causes will often spare the forehead as these muscles receive fibres from both facial nerve nuclei.

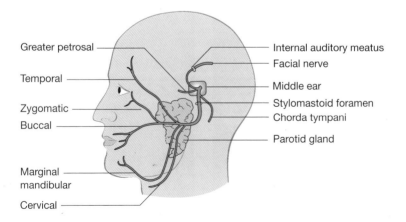

Figure 15.1 Facial nerve anatomy.

Diseases of the Ear, Nose and Throat Lecture Notes, Eleventh edition. Ray Clarke. © 2014 John Wiley & Sons Ltd. Published 2014 by John Wiley & Sons, Ltd.

Table 15.1 Common causes of facial nerve paralysis

Supranuclear and nuclear (upper motor neurone)
- Vascular lesions, e.g. stroke
- Intracranial tumours
- Multiple sclerosis

Infranuclear (lower motor neurone)
- 'Bell's palsy'
- Trauma (birth injury, fractured temporal bone, surgical)
- Tumours (parotid tumours, acoustic neuroma, malignant disease of the middle ear)
- Middle ear suppuration (acute or chronic otitis media)
- 'Ramsay Hunt' syndrome
- Guillain–Barré syndrome
- Sarcoidosis

Clinical diagnosis

The patient presents with weakness of the facial muscles, difficulty in clearing food from inside the cheek, or drooling from one side of the mouth. Facial asymmetry is accentuated by asking the patient to attempt to close the eyes tightly, show the teeth or whistle (Fig. 15.2).

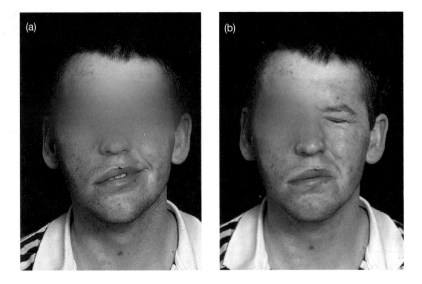

Figure 15.2 Post-traumatic right facial palsy. Shown at rest (a) and on attempted eye closure (b).

Involuntary movements (e.g. smiling) may be retained even in the lower face. A careful history and aural and neurological examination are essential. Sparing of the forehead suggests a supranuclear pathology. Impaired taste implies the lesion is above the origin of the chorda tympani; reduction of tear production (lacrimation) suggests the lesion is above the geniculate ganglion where the superficial petrosal nerve arises.

Bell's palsy (idiopathic facial paralysis)

Bell's palsy is a lower motor neurone facial palsy of unknown cause, but thought to be viral. Bell's palsy may be complete or incomplete; the more severe the palsy, the worse the prognosis. In practice, full recovery may be expected in over 90% of cases. The remainder may develop persistent paraylsis and other complications including ectropion (weakness of the muscles of the lower eyelid causing persistent overflow of tears) or an aberrant sequence of movements of the face (synkinesis).

Assessment and investigations

- CT or MRI scanning may be needed if the symptoms persist or a specific cause (i.e. other than Bell's palsy) is suspected.
- Electrodiagnosis is used in the assessment of the degree of involvement of the nerve and includes nerve conduction tests and electromyography. These tests are done in a specialist centre and be invaluable in predicting prognosis.

Management of Bell's palsy

- Treatment of Bell's palsy should be commenced as soon as possible.
- Prednisolone given orally is the treatment of choice, but it must commence in the first 72 hours. In an adult, start with 25 mgs twice daily for up to ten days.
- Be vigilant about eye care. The protective blink reflex may be lost and the cornea exposed, especially at night. An eyepad, a tape over the eyelids at night or in persistent cases a 'tarsorrhaphy' (surgical approximation of the eyelids) may be needed.
- Antivirals such as acyclovir seem to offer little benefit.
- Persistent facial palsy warrants referral and thorough investigation, including CT or MRI scanning.

Ramsay Hunt syndrome

This is due to herpes zoster infection of the geniculate ganglion, affecting more rarely the glossopharyngeal (IX) and vagus (X) nerves and, very occasionally, the trigeminal (V), abducens (VI) or hypoglossal (XII) nerves. The patient is usually elderly, and severe pain precedes the facial palsy. The patient often has vertigo, and the hearing is impaired. The characteristic clinical feature is a vesicular eruption in the ear (sometimes on the tongue and palate). Recovery of facial nerve function is much less likely than in Bell's palsy.

Prompt treatment with acyclovir given orally may improve the prognosis and reduce post-herpetic neuralgia.

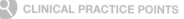

 CLINICAL PRACTICE POINTS

- Do not make a diagnosis of Bell's palsy until you have excluded other causes. If recovery does not commence in 6 weeks, reconsider the diagnosis.
- Facial palsy in acute or chronic otitis media requires immediate expert advice. Refer for urgent surgical advice

Go to **www.lecturenoteseries.com/ENT** to test yourself using the interactive MCQs.

Part 2

The nose and sinuses

16

Clinical examination of the nose and nasopharynx

Applied basic science

The nose is made up of a framework of bone and cartilage, lined with skin on the outside and with mucosa on the inside (Fig. 16.1). The nasal mucosa is lined for the most part with ciliated columnar epithelium except for a small area of highly specialized olfactory mucosa, which is receptive to scents and odours and communicates with the olfactory nerve. The largest of the cartilages that makes up the nose is the septal cartilage, dividing the nasal cavity in two. The anterior part of the nose is termed the nasal vestibule. The posterior nasal apertures are the choanae. These open to the upper part of the pharynx – the nasopharynx.

The lateral wall of the nose is contoured with three bony swellings, covered with mucosa, projecting into the nasal cavity. These are the turbinates, which can become engorged and swollen when inflamed- 'rhinitis'.

Functions of the nose

- A conduit for the passage of air-the first part of the respiratory tract.
- Part of the respiratory defence against infection.
- Warms and humidifies inspired air.
- Olfaction.

Diseases of the Ear, Nose and Throat Lecture Notes, Eleventh edition. Ray Clarke. © 2014 John Wiley & Sons Ltd.
Published 2014 by John Wiley & Sons, Ltd.

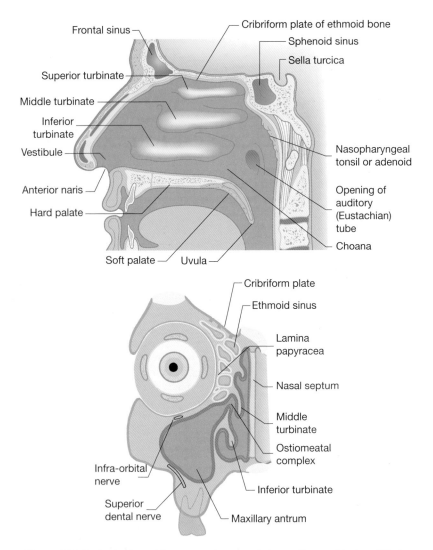

Figure 16.1 Basic structure of the nose and paranasal sinuses. Source: Munir and Clarke 2013. *Ear, Nose and Throat at a Glance*. With permission of John Wiley & Sons Ltd.

The sinuses

The paranasal sinuses are a series of air-filled cavities that communicate directly with the nose. They are lined with nasal mucosa and are subject to the same diseases as the nose itself – notably inflammatory processes. Hence the term 'rhinosinusitis' is more accurate than 'sinusitis'.

The maxillary sinus or 'antrum' is the largest of the sinuses with a capacity in the adult of approximately 15 mL. The orbit lies above and the hard palate with the roots of the second premolar and the first two molar teeth forms the floor. Medially the antrum is separated from the nose by the lateral nasal wall made up of the middle and inferior turbinate bones, each with a corresponding recess or 'meatus' below it (Fig. 16.1).

The ethmoidal sinuses form a honeycomb of air cells between the 'lamina papyracea' or thin bone at the medial wall of the orbit and the upper part of the nose. An upward extension forms the fronto-nasal duct draining the frontal sinus. The frontal sinus is within the frontal bone in the forehead and the sphenoidal sinus is in the midline within the sphenoid bone behind the nose.

The openings of the sinuses under the middle turbinate form the ostiomeatal complex. It is now recognized that abnormality of this area leads to failure of sinus drainage and thence to sinusitis. Abnormalities may be structural, as with a large aerated cell blocking the ostial openings. Functional anomalies such as oedema, allergy or polyp formation can also obstruct the ostiomeatal complex.

Examination of the nose

Illumination and inspection

The first requirement is adequate lighting. Use a headlight, an endoscope or a head-mirror to reflect light from an adjustable strong light source. All of these take some training and experience to use well. A bright torch or better still an auriscope with the largest speculum that will fit into the nasal cavity provides a good alternative (Fig. 16.2).

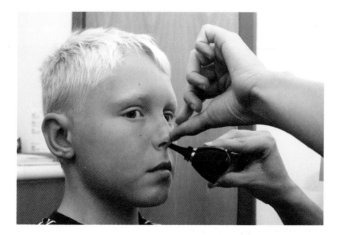

Figure 16.2 Using an aural speculum to inspect the nasal cavity. Note the direction of view.

First inspect the exterior of the nose. Look for asymmetry of the nasal bones and gently lift the nasal tip to look for any deviation of the septum and any evidence of inflammation of the skin around the entrance to the nasal cavity (vestibule).

The nasal airway

Now assess the nasal airway. You can do this by gently occluding one nostril at a time and asking the patient to breathe in through the other side, or by holding a cool polished surface such as a metal tongue depressor below the nostrils. The areas of condensation from each side of the nose can be compared.

Anterior rhinoscopy and nasendoscopy

Most students are unaware of the interior dimensions and relations of the nose, which extends horizontally backwards for 65–76 mm to the posterior nasal apertures or 'choanae'. Remember that the interior of the nose is much more horizontal than most students think and that the nasal mucosa is very sensitive! When you look in remember to look 'back' rather than 'up' (Fig. 16.2). The inside of the nose may be obscured by mucosal oedema or septal deviations. A good way to test the patency of the nasal airway especially in children, is to use a cold metal spatula under the nostrils to see the condensation pattern of expired air (Fig. 16.3).

ENT surgeons will sometimes use a Thudicum's speculum (Fig. 16.4), which is introduced gently into the nose. In children, a speculum is often not necessary as an adequate view can be obtained by lifting the nasal tip with the thumb.

Nasal endoscopes have improved greatly in recent years and rigid endoscopy is now the standard way to inspect the interior of the nose. The instrument is introduced through the nose and the nose and nasopharynx (postnasal space) can be easily seen, allowing photography and simultaneous viewing by an observer.

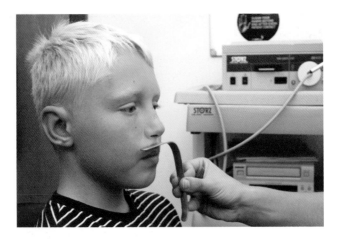

Figure 16.3 Assessing the nasal airway using a metal tongue depressor.

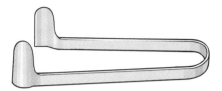

Figure 16.4 Thudicum's speculum.

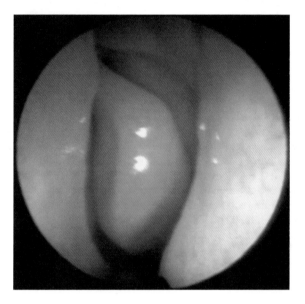

Figure 16.5 The appearance of the normal nose showing the inferior turbinate attached to the lateral nasal wall (courtesy of T.J. Woolford).

On looking into the nose the anterior septum and inferior turbinates are easily seen (Fig. 16.5). It is a common error to mistake the turbinates for a nasal polyp. Turbinates are sensitive, and are attached to the lateral nasal wall. A polyp is often greyish, translucent and insensitive to touch.

🔍 CLINICAL PRACTICE POINT

- An auriscope with a large speculum provides a good view of the inside of the nose.

 Go to **www.lecturenoteseries.com/ENT** to test yourself using the interactive MCQs.

17

The nasal septum

✓ The nasal septum is made up of bone and cartilage. It can be **deviated,
  perforated,** or **collapsed**.

Septal deviation

The nasal septum is rarely exactly in the midline (Fig. 17.1). Minor deviations are
normal and cause no symptoms. Marked deviation will cause nasal airway obstruction and may contribute to sino-nasal pathology by obstructing the normal sinus
drainage pathways. Septal deviation can be corrected by surgery, with excellent
results.

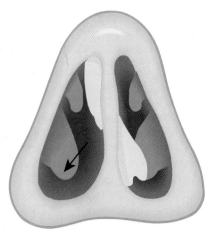

Figure 17.1 'S'-shaped deviation of the nasal septum with hypertrophy of the right
middle turbinate (arrowed).

Diseases of the Ear, Nose and Throat Lecture Notes, Eleventh edition. Ray Clarke. © 2014 John Wiley & Sons Ltd.
Published 2014 by John Wiley & Sons, Ltd.

Aetiology

Most cases of deviated nasal septum (DNS) result from trauma, either recent or long forgotten, perhaps during birth. 'Buckling' in children may become more pronounced as the septum grows. Nasal surgery, including cosmetic surgery, can cause septal deviation.

Effects

- Nasal obstruction – may be unilateral or bilateral.
- Recurrent sinus infection due to impairment of sinus ventilation by the displaced septum. The middle turbinate on the concave side of the septum may hypertrophy and interfere with sinus ventilation.
- Severe deviation is apparent on looking at the nose and septal surgery is an important component of aesthetic nasal surgery (septorhinoplasty).
- Can cause facial pain but this is rare.
- Otitis media. DNS may impair the ability to equalize middle-ear pressure.
- Nosebleeds – a sharp spur can be a focus for epistaxis (Fig. 17.2).

Treatment

- If symptoms are minimal and there is only a minor degree of deviation, no treatment is needed. Septal deviations are often found in patients with allergic rhinitis. Treat the rhinitis rather than the septal deviation. Where symptoms are more severe correction of the septal deformity is justified (though never essential).

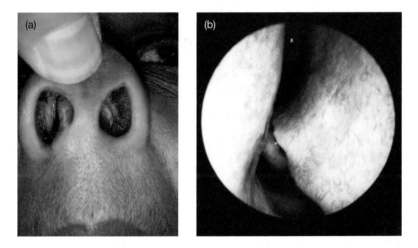

Figure 17.2 (a) Deviated nasal septum and (b) endoscopic view.

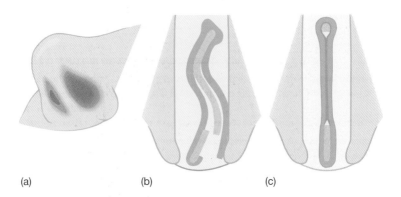

(a)   (b)   (c)

Figure 17.3 Nasal septal surgery (septoplasty). (a) Incision through the muco-perichondrium. (b) Elevation of muco-perichondrial flaps on either side of the septal skeleton. (c) The displaced cartilage and bone have been resected, allowing the septum to resume a midline position.

- Surgery involves elevating mucosal flaps from the septal cartilage and resecting part of the deviated cartilage before replacing it in the midline (septoplasty; Fig. 17.3).
- Septal surgery should be undertaken with caution if at all in children as it may interfere with the growth of the mid-face.

Septal perforation (Fig. 17.4)

Aetiology

Perforation of the nasal septum may result from the following conditions:

- Nasal surgery.
- Trauma including repeated nose-picking.
- Chronic inflammation, e.g. nasal granulomatosis, syphilis.
- Inhalation of fumes, e.g. chrome salts.
- Cocaine.
- Carcinoma.

Effects

Many septal perforations cause no trouble. They may give rise to epistaxis and crusting or rarely whistling on inspiration or expiration. A perforation is readily seen and often has unhealthy edges covered with large crusts.

Nasal septum ⎯⎤   ⎡⎯ Septal perforation

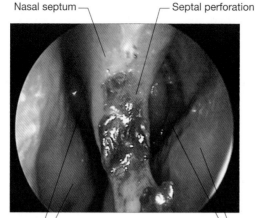

Right inferior and / /   \ \ Left inferior and
middle turbinates   middle turbinates

Figure 17.4 Nasal septal perforation. Source: Munir and Clarke 2013. *Ear, Nose and Throat at a Glance*. Reproduced with permission of Nazia Munir and Ray Clarke.

Treatment

- Septal perforations are very difficult to repair.
- Nasal douching with saline or bicarbonate solution reduces crusting around the edge of the defect.
- Antiseptic cream will help control infection. Be careful with creams based on peanut oil, e.g. Naseptin TM, as they can cause severe reactions in patients with peanut allergy.
- A self-retaining double-flanged silastic button can be inserted into the perforation.
- If crusting and bleeding remain a problem, the perforation can be closed surgically.

Septal collapse (saddle nose) (Fig. 17.5)

The cartilaginous septum can necrose following **repeated trauma**, an untreated nasal **septal haematoma**, or after extensive **nasal surgery**. Some **chronic inflammatory conditions**, e.g. nasal granulomatosis, syphilis, and tuberculosis can cause septal necrosis with 'saddling'. Patients complain of the aesthetic deformity and may also get very troublesome nasal obstruction. Treatment is difficult and may require extensive surgery to both the cartilage and the nasal bones– 'augmentation septorhinoplasty'.

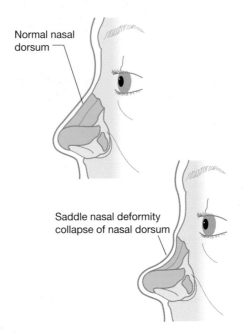

Normal nasal dorsum

Saddle nasal deformity collapse of nasal dorsum

Figure 17.5 Saddle nose. Source: Munir and Clarke 2013. *Ear, Nose and Throat at a Glance*. With permission of John Wiley & Sons Ltd.

> ### CLINICAL PRACTICE POINT
> • Minor deviations of the nasal septum are normal. If the patient has nasal symptoms, rhinitis is a far more common cause. Treat it first.

Nasal septal perforation may be asymptomatic and need no treatment.

 Go to **www.lecturenoteseries.com/ENT** to test yourself using the interactive MCQs.

18

Acute nose and sinus infections

Acute coryza

The common cold is the result of viral infection but secondary bacterial infection may supervene. It is self-limiting and no treatment is required other than an antipyretic, such as paracetamol. Discourage the prolonged use (more than 5 days) of vasoconstrictor nose drops owing to their harmful effect on the nasal mucosa (**rhinitis medicamentosa**). Many patients use menthol inhalations, systemic decongestants and a variety of cough linctus preparations, and find these helpful in controlling symptoms, but evidence of any sustained benefit is weak.

Nasal vestibulitis

Both children and adults may be carriers of pyogenic staphylococci, which can produce infection of the skin of the nasal vestibule. The site becomes sore, fissured and crusted. Treatment consists of topical antibiotic/antiseptic ointment. Consider systemic flucloxacillin in more severe cases. In children with persistent vestibulitis look for a nasal foreign body.

Furunculosis

An abscess in a nasal hair follicle is rare but must be treated seriously as it can spread rapidly and lead to cavernous sinus thrombosis and meningitis. The tip of the nose becomes red, tense and painful. Give systemic antibiotics without delay. Drainage may be necessary but should be deferred until the patient has had adequate antibiotic treatment for 24 h. In recurrent cases, exclude immunodeficiency.

Diseases of the Ear, Nose and Throat Lecture Notes, Eleventh edition. Ray Clarke. © 2014 John Wiley & Sons Ltd. Published 2014 by John Wiley & Sons, Ltd.

Acute sinus infection

Aetiology

Most cases of acute sinusitis are secondary to acute viral illness, e.g. coryza, which causes nasal mucosal oedema and interferes with ventilation and mucous clearance from the sinuses. The paranasal sinuses become infected as part of generalized infection of the nose and sinus mucosa – **rhinosinusitis**. Usually more than one sinus is involved (*pan-sinusitis*; Fig. 18.1). Bacterial infection supervenes causing purulent rhinorrhoea. The causative organisms are usually pyogenic, e.g. *Streptococcus pneumoniae, Haemophilus influenzae* or *Staphylococcus pyogenes*. Anaerobes may be involved especially in dental infections.

Many patients have a background of rhinitis, often allergic in origin, which predisposes them to episodes of ostiomeatal complex obstruction and sinus infection.

In about 10% of cases of maxillary sinusitis the infection is dental in origin and has spread from the upper molars or premolars. Occasionally, infection follows

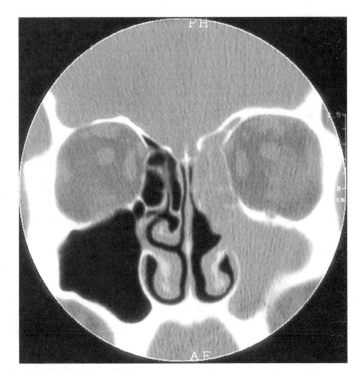

Figure 18.1 Coronal CT scan showing left-sided ethmoidal and maxillary sinusitis.

the entry of infected material, e.g. after diving – water is forced through the ostium into the sinus.

Clinical features

- Nasal obstruction.
- Nasal discharge (rhinorhoea).
- A feeling of 'congestion' in the nose and face.
- Facial pain. In maxillary sinusitis the pain is mainly over the cheeks; ethmoidal and frontal sinusitis cause periorbital pain and headache, and sphenoidal sinusitis causes severe deep-seated headache.
- Pyrexial illness.
- Mucopus in the nose.
- Tenderness over the involved sinuses.
- Cheek swelling may indicate a dental abscess.

The diagnosis should be made clinically. Acute sinusitis typically resolves but may recur.

X-rays are not needed but CT scanning can be very helpful if there are complications.

Treatment

- **Adequate analgesia**
- **Antibiotics**. If the nasal discharge is mucopurulent, Cefaclor is a useful first-line.
- **Vasoconstrictor** nose drops, such as 1% ephedrine or 0.05% oxymetazoline, will aid drainage of the sinus. Use these sparingly and only for short periods (3–5 days is enough).
- **Surgery:** If the ostiomeatal complex is completely obstructed there may be severe pain due to retained pus (empyaema). Initial treatment is medical but surgery may be necessary. Drainage of the sinuses is nowadays by endoscopic surgery of the ostiomeatal area under the middle turbinate – functional endoscopic sinus surgery (FESS). Developments in endoscopic instruments now allow inspection of the sinus ostia and interior of the paranasal sinuses. Ostial enlargement and removal of polyps and cysts can be performed. The ostiomeatal complex under the middle turbinate is opened up. This allows a more 'physiological' drainage of the antrum than was possible before the development of endoscopic endonasal surgery and 'antral washout' – insertion of a trochar into the antrum via the nasal cavity with aspiration of the contents of the antrum – is now rarely performed. Apiration of an empyaema by whatever means brings dramatic relief.

Refer immediately if you suspect complications- e.g. severe headache, neurological changes or eye changes

Complications of acute rhinosinusitis

Complications may arise if the infection spreads beyond the bony walls of the sinuses (Fig. 18.2). These are rare in Western communities but still a significant cause of morbidity and mortality worldwide. Beware of the patient with sinusitis who develops severe headache, swinging pyrexia or neurological signs:

- Orbital complications (cellulitis or abscess) are characterized by marked oedema of the eyelids, diplopia, redness and swelling of the conjunctiva (chemosis). Proptosis indicates severe orbital involvement. Commence intravenous antibiotics immediately and ask for an urgent ENT opinion. Resolution usually follows intensive antibiotic therapy but surgical drainage is required urgently if there is any change in vision. Loss of colour discrimination is an early sign of impending visual loss.
- Meningitis, extradural and subdural abscesses may occur and should be treated as neurosurgical emergencies.
- Cerebral abscess (frontal lobe). Any patient with a history of recent frontal sinus infection headaches or who exhibits any abnormality of behaviour should be suspected of a frontal lobe abscess.
- Osteomyelitis of the frontal bone is characterized by persistent headache and oedema of the scalp in the vicinity of the frontal sinus. X-ray signs are late, and by the time they become apparent osteomyelitis is well established. Intensive antibiotic therapy combined with removal of diseased bone is necessary.
- Cavernous sinus thrombosis is very rare. Proptosis, chemosis (corneal oedema) and ophthalmoplegia characterize this dangerous complication (Fig. 18.3).
- Poor sinus drainage can cause a bony swelling as secretions build up in the obstructed sinus- 'mucocoele'. (Fig. 18.4) Treatment is surgical.

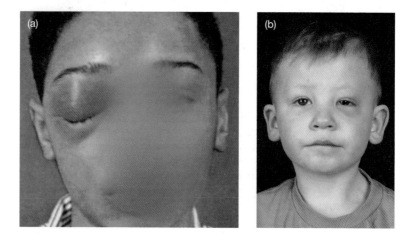

Figure 18.2 (a) Orbital cellulitis. (b) Resolving orbital cellulitis.

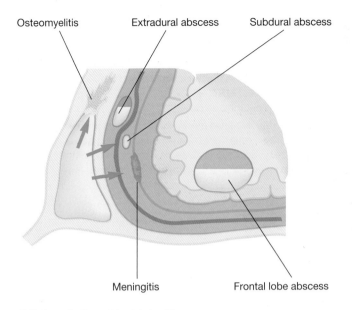

Figure 18.3 Complications of frontal sinusitis.

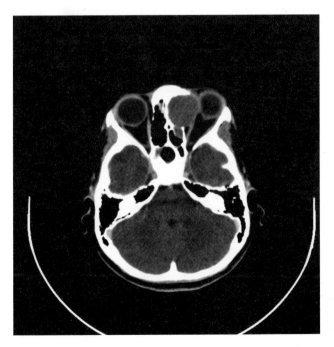

Figure 18.4 Fronto-ethmoidal mucocoele.

CLINICAL PRACTICE POINTS

- Assume a child with a unilateral nasal discharge has a nasal foreign body.
- Most cases of sinusitis resolve but complications can be devastating. Beware of the sinusitis patient with severe headache, suspected neurological signs or orbital swelling.
- Many patients suffer repeated misery due to frequent and recurrent episodes of rhinosinusitis. Refer to an ENT surgeon so that anatomical abnormalities, e.g. nasal septal deviations, ostiomeatal complex anomalies, and ciliary and immunological function can be checked.

Go to **www.lecturenoteseries.com/ENT** to test yourself using the interactive MCQs.

19

Tumours of the nose, sinuses and nasopharynx

✓ Nasal and sinus tumours are typically squamous cell carcinomas (SCC) and metastasize to the lymph nodes of the neck. They are rare, and often not diagnosed until they have spread to surrounding structures.

Aetiology

Tobacco and alcohol are important aetiological factors. Men are more commonly affected. One of the risk factors for development of **adenocarcinoma** of the maxillary antrum is exposure to the resins produced by hardwoods and woodworkers are at increased risk. Take a careful occupational history. Nasopharyngeal Carcinoma (NPC) is rare in Europe but relatively common in the Far East in general and in southern China in particular. The Epstein–Barr virus plays a role in the aetiology of nasopharyngeal malignancy. Dietary factors – salted fish and meats – may partly explain the increased risk in South China but genetic factors are important as well.

Carcinoma of the maxillary and ethmoidal sinuses

Clinical features

In its earliest stages these tumours cause no symptoms. Blood-stained nasal discharge and increasing unilateral nasal obstruction should raise suspicion.

Diseases of the Ear, Nose and Throat Lecture Notes, Eleventh edition. Ray Clarke. © 2014 John Wiley & Sons Ltd.
Published 2014 by John Wiley & Sons, Ltd.

Late features are sadly often the presenting features and include:

- Unilateral facial swelling.
- Swelling or ulceration of the gums or palate.
- Epiphora, owing to involvement of the nasolacrimal duct.
- Proptosis and diplopia, due to involvement of the floor of the orbit.
- Pain – commonly in the cheek, but may be referred to the ear, head or jaw
- Metastatic neck nodes

Malignant disease of the nasopharynx

Clinical features

- Nasal obstruction and blood-stained nasal discharge.
- Patients may present with conductive deafness. Otitis media with effusion results from Eustachian tube obstruction.
- Invasion of the skull base causes involvement of various cranial nerves, especially nerves V (paraesthesia in the face and corneal anaesthesia), VI (ophthalmoplegia), IX (pain in the throat, loss of gag reflex), X (hoarseness) and XII (abnormal tongue movement).
- Enlarged cervical nodes – may be bilateral.

Other tumours of the nasal region (Fig. 19.1)

Osteomata

Osteomata are benign bony tumours usually in the frontal and ethmoidal sinuses. They are slow-growing and cause few symptoms but may eventually call for surgical removal.

Nasopharyngeal angiofibroma

Nasopharyngeal angiofibroma is a rare benign tumour of adolescent boys. It presents as epistaxis and nasal obstruction, and is usually easily visible by posterior rhinoscopy. Being highly vascular, the tumour is locally destructive and extends into the surrounding structures. Diagnosis is confirmed by MR scanning.

Malignant granuloma

Though not truly neoplastic, malignant granuloma is a sinister condition characterized by progressive ulceration of the nose and neighbouring structures. This is probably a variant of lymphoma.

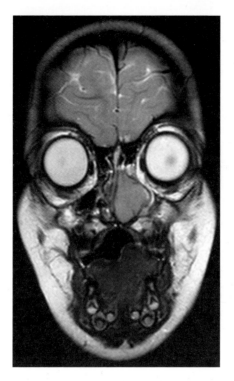

Figure 19.1 MRI scan of a left-sided nasal mass. Histology confirmed a non-Hodgkin's lymphoma.

Malignant melanoma

Malignant melanoma is fortunately rare in the nose and sinuses. Treatment is by radical surgery but the prognosis is extremely poor.

Treatment of nasal and sinus tumours

- Treatment of nasopharyngeal cancer is mainly by radiotherapy. Surgery may be needed for late disease and for neck metastases.
- Antro-ethmoidal tumours may be too far advanced for curative treatment at presentation. A combination of surgery and radiotherapy offers the best chance. Total maxillectomy (with exenteration of the orbit if involved) may be needed. This results in a large defect in the hard palate, for which a modified upper denture with an obturator is provided. Even with radical treatment, nasal sinus carcinoma has a poor prognosis, with only about 30% of patients surviving to 5 years.
- Angiofibroma is treated by surgical removal with a good prognosis.

CLINICAL PRACTICE POINTS

- NPC can present with unilateral deafness, enlarged cervical nodes or cranial nerve palsies. Maintain a high index of suspicion, especially in Chinese patients.
- Paranasal sinus and post-nasal space tumours present late.

Go to **www.lecturenoteseries.com/ENT** to test yourself using the interactive MCQs.

20

Rhinitis and nasal polyps

Rhinitis

Rhinitis refers to inflammatory changes in the nasal mucosa. As the nasal mucosa is continuous over the nose and sinuses, there is nearly always some inflammatory change in the sinuses as well. Hence **Rhinisinusitis** is a better term.

Acute nose and sinus infections are dealt with in Chapter 18. Continuing inflammatory change or repeated episodes of recurrent rhinosinusitis so that episodes merge one with the other are common – **Chronic Rhinosinusitis (CR)**. Continuing mucosal inflammation causes polypoid swelling of the nasal lining (**Nasal Polyps,** hence the close association between **Chronic Rhinosinusitis** and **Nasal Polyps (CRNP))**. The misery brought about by inflammation of the nose is one of the commonest reasons for patients to consult a GP or ENT surgeon. The adverse effect on quality of life is considerable, and often underestimated. Many patients self-medicate, miss time from work or school, and may develop severe asthma as part of a general pattern of respiratory tract allergy.

Prevalence and trends

Rhinosinusitis is on the increase and may affect more than a quarter of the population, particularly in the developed world. The main allergens are pollens, troublesome in the spring and early summer (seasonal allergic rhinitis or 'hay fever'), the ubiquitous house-dust mite which lives on desquamated human skin (Fig. 20.1), animal dander (e.g. from cats or dogs) and, less often, mould spores which are particularly active in autumn. The reasons for this increase are unclear but suggestions include a decreased exposure to infections in childhood so that the immune system is less thoroughly stimulated in early life, air pollution and dietary changes.

Diseases of the Ear, Nose and Throat Lecture Notes, Eleventh edition. Ray Clarke. © 2014 John Wiley & Sons Ltd. Published 2014 by John Wiley & Sons, Ltd.

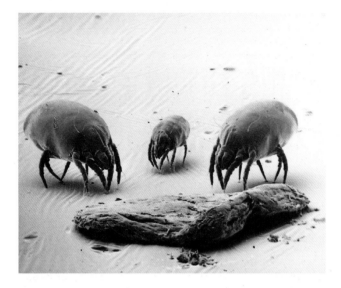

Figure 20.1 Scanning electron micrograph of house-dust mites and a human squame. (Crown copyright reproduced courtesy of Dr D.A. Griffiths, Slough Laboratory, Slough.)

Aetiology and classification of rhinitis

Allergy is a key cause of mucosal inflammation (Allergic Rhinitis AR) and is the commonest initiating pathology. Infection may coexist, or may complicate an existing allergic rhinosinusitis. Some cases are due to neither allergy nor infection (nonallergic, non-infectious rhinitis). Box 20.1 shows some of the common causes of rhinosinusitis.

Box 20.1 Common causes of chronic rhinosinusitis (CRS)

- **Allergic rhinitis (AR)** – allergens include pollens, weeds, house dust mite, moulds, animal dander- e.g. cats and dogs
- **Infectious rhinitis**
  Hormonal, e.g. rhinitis of pregnancy, hypothyroidism.
  Drug induced, e.g. beta-blockers, contraceptive pill.
- **Occupational rhinitis** – some chemicals and fumes can be highly irritant to the nasal mucosa.
- **Neurogenic or 'vasomotor' rhinitis** – the term 'neurogenic rhinitis' is not often used nowadays and it probably refers to normal variation in the state of engorgement of the nasal mucosa – the nasal cycle. For some patients, this

continuing flux in the state of filling of the nasal vasculature causes troublesome nasal obstruction and the term 'vasomotor rhinitis' is used. A trial of intranasal steroids may be helpful. These patients should be discouraged from repeated use of nasal decongestants due to the risk of rhinitis medicamentosa.

- **Rhinitis medicamentosa** – excessive use of nasal decongestants causes rebound nasal congestion. Treatment is to stop the drops or sprays.
- **Atrophic rhinitis** – characterized by drying and crusting of the nose. It can follow extensive nasal surgery, radiotherapy or Sjögren's syndrome.
- **Senile rhinitis** – elderly patients may develop troublesome rhinorrhoea, causing a 'drip' at the end of the nose. This often responds well to ipratroprium bromide, an atropine-like spray.

Pathogenesis of allergic rhinitis

The nasal mucosa is at the entrance to the respiratory tract. It is made up of ciliated epithelium and produces a mucus blanket which helps protect the airway from inspired pollutants, allergens and infective agents. The epithelium is continuous with that of the rest of the respiratory system and is subject to much the same pathologies.

The allergen induces production of IgE antibodies which on subsequent exposure bind with the allergen to form antigen–antibody complexes. These complexes then attach to mast cells in the nasal epithelium, causing the cells to rupture and release inflammatory mediators including histamine (Type 1 allergic response). An intense local inflammatory reaction ensues with oedema and secretion of mucus. The nose may now become sensitive to irritants in inspired air, so that the slightest stimulus will cause symptoms to recur.

Allergic rhinitis primarily occurs in atopic individuals. **Atopy** is a general increased sensitivity to the production of Immunoglobulin E in response to small amounts of allergens-typically specific proteins. Atopic people may develop both rhinitis and asthma (**'sneezles and wheezles'**) and they often have a strong family history of these disorders and of eczema.

Clinical features

Diagnosis is clinical. You don't usually need X-rays or scans. The main symptoms are:

- a feeling of nasal congestion;
- nasal airflow obstruction;
- rhinorrhoea or a watery nasal discharge;
- sneezing;
- reduced or absent sense of smell (hyposmia or anosmia).

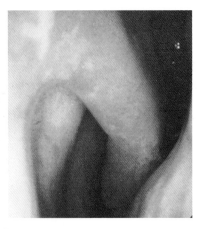

Figure 20.2 Nasal endoscopy

Take a careful history and enquire particularly about other manifestations of allergy, e.g. eczema and asthma. The association with asthma is very strong – not only can they coexist but AR can make asthma worse – remember Allergic Rhinitis and its Impact on Asthma (**ARIA**). Enquire about family history.

Examine the nose and look at the skin for evidence of a crease – 'allergic crease' – just above the tip. This is due to the patient rubbing the nose to relieve itching. Look for redness or swelling of the mucosa – particularly the turbinates – and a mucoid discharge. Check for structural anomalies such a septal deviation or nasal polyps, but even if these are noted it is wise to treat the rhinitis. Investigations are not usually needed but sensitivity tests for specific allergens – 'skin prick tests' – may help to direct allergen avoidance therapy.

Nasal endoscopy will show oedema and often polypoid change (Fig. 20.2).

Nasal polyps

Nasal polyps are composed of swollen and oedematous nasal mucosal tissues. They can cause complete nasal obstruction. Nasal polyposis will usually be accompanied by evidence of widespread mucosal disease throughout the sinuses when seen on a CT scan (Fig. 20.3) but the diagnosis is clinical and scans are usually only needed to help plan surgery.

Polyps are yellowish-grey, smooth and moist (Fig. 20.4). They are pedunculated and move on gentle probing although they are insensitive, unlike the inferior turbinate. It is easy to see the inferior turbinate and mistake it for a polyp – do not be caught out.

Nasal polyps may be a feature of long-standing rhinitis of any cause. They are thought to arise mainly from the mucosa of the ethmoid sinuses which gradually

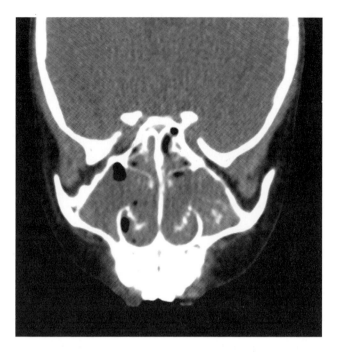

Figure 20.3 Scan showing extensive pansinusits and nasal polyps.

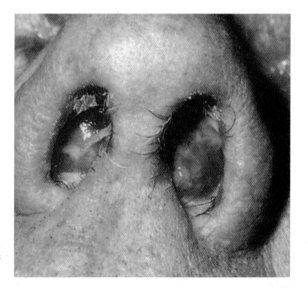

Figure 20.4 Multiple ethmoidal polyps.

swells until it projects into the nose, giving the polyps a pedunculated appearance. Histologically, nasal polyps consist of a loose oedematous stroma infiltrated by inflammatory lymphocytes and eosinophils and covered by respiratory epithelium. Nasal polyposis is usually a mucosal disease and presents in both the nostrils. Beware of unilateral polyps, which may represent a neoplastic lesion. More often, a unilateral polyp is an 'antrochoanal' polyp. This is usually solitary and benign, arising within the maxillary antrum, extruding through the ostium and presenting as a smooth swelling in the nasopharynx. Such a polyp may extend below the soft palate and be several centimetres in length. Treatment is surgical removal. Beware of nasal polyps in children. Think of cystic fibrosis or in a newborn baby a nasal glioma or a nasal encephalocele.

Differential diagnosis of CRS/NP

- **Adenoidal hypertrophy** can cause nasal obstruction and discoloured nasal secretions.
- **Nasal septal deviation** alone can also cause nasal symptoms but will often co-exist with rhinitis.
- A **foreign body** in the nose may go undetected and should be thought of especially with unilateral discharge in a child.
- **Cystic fibrosis** and **primary ciliary dyskinesia** are both rare but can present with rhinosinusitis-like symptoms.
- A **unilateral nasal 'polyp'** may be a tumour
- Very rarely indeed a watery nasal discharge may be cerebrospinal fluid (**CSF rhinorrhoea**), particularly after a head injury or nasal surgery that has breached the meninges.

Treatment

Try medical treatment first. Surgery is very much a last resort.

- Allergen avoidance measures include minimizing contact with house-dust or pollens.
- Systemic or intranasal antihistamines help control symptoms.
- Intranasal steroids – the mainstay of treatment.
- Systemic antibiotics for infection – may need a prolonged or repeated course.
- Sodium chromoglycate – stabilizes mast cells. Not so widely used now as nasal steroids have improved with less systemic absorption.
- Nasal decongestants – use sparingly and briefly if at all.
- Oral leukotriene receptor antagonists *(Montelukast)* may have a role but these are more commonly prescribed for severe asthma.

Small nasal polyps will reduce in size in reponse to steroids – '**medical polypectomy**'. Both topical and systemic treatment can be combined, but this is best done under the supervision of an ENT surgeon, and if you see or suspect nasal polyps it is best to refer the patient to a specialist clinic. Figure 20.5 is a useful algorithm to guide the medical management of rhinosinusitis.

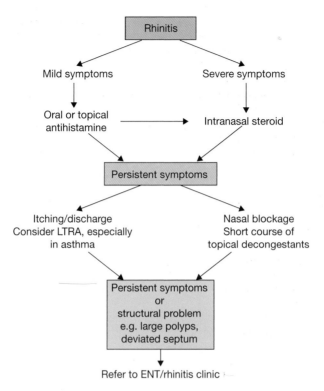

LTRA = Leukotrine receptor antagonist
- Consider a course of antibiotics if there is evidence of active nose or sinus infection.
- Consider a short course of systemic steroids if symptoms are severe or to shrink nasal polyps.

Figure 20.5 Primary care management of rhinitis. If in doubt, refer to an ENT/rhinitis clinic.

Surgery

Nasal polypectomy may be needed. Persistent symptoms despite intensive medical treatment may warrant surgery to improve sinus drainage – **Functional Endoscopic Sinus Surgery (FESS)** – or to improve the airway. If the patient has a severe nasal septal deviation then **septal surgery** may be considered. Surgery to reduce the size of the inferior turbinates was popular in the past but is now rarely needed.

CLINICAL PRACTICE POINTS

- Rhinitis – particularly due to allergy – is on the increase.
- Rhinosinusitis causes a lot of morbidity and is under-recognized.
- An intranasal steroid is a good first-line treatment for rhinitis of any cause.
- Beware of unilateral nasal polyps and polyps in children.

Go to **www.lecturenoteseries.com/ENT** to test yourself using the interactive MCQs.

21

Facial plastic surgery

✓ ENT surgeons are increasingly involved in surgery of the face.

Facial skin cancers

Many benign skin lesions – e.g. keratosis, kerato-acanthoma, benign pigmented lesions – can present on the face but it is wise to be vigilant and refer early if you have any concerns. Cutaneous cancers of the scalp and face are the most common malignancies of any part of the body. They present typically in fair-skinned people exposed to sunlight and are more common in the elderly. Prognosis with early detection is excellent.

Types of facial skin cancer

Basal Cell Carcinoma (BCC)

There are a number of different clinical types but typically they grow slowly and ulcerate at the centre (Figs 21.1 and 21.2). The central ulcer is surrounded by a pearly-looking rolled edge that looks as if it has been nibbled, hence the older term 'rodent ulcer'. Although they don't tend to metastasize, these tumours are locally aggressive and can cause extensive soft tissue destruction, eventually eroding into the facial bones.

Squamous Cell Carcinoma (SCC)

This is less common and does not have the typically 'rolled edge' of a BCC (Fig. 21.3). SCCs are much more aggressive, spread to regional lymph nodes and may need extensive surgery. Both SCCs and BCCs may be multiple.

Malignant melanoma

This is by far the most aggressive of the skin cancers that affect the face (Fig. 21.4). It usually – but not always – arises from an existing pigmented lesion. Be vigilant about seeking advice if pigmented skin lesions change.

Diseases of the Ear, Nose and Throat Lecture Notes, Eleventh edition. Ray Clarke. © 2014 John Wiley & Sons Ltd. Published 2014 by John Wiley & Sons, Ltd.

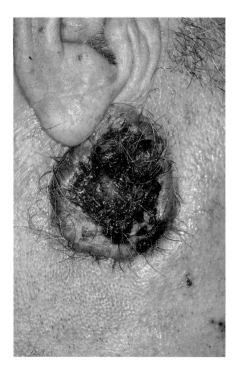

Figure 21.1 Basal cell carcinoma ('rodent ulcer') of the skin of the cheek. Note the rolled edges. (Courtesy of Mr David Richardson, FRCS, Liverpool.)

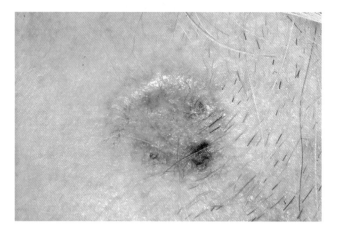

Figure 21.2 Early basal cell carcinoma. (Courtesy of Mr David Richardson, FRCS, Liverpool.)

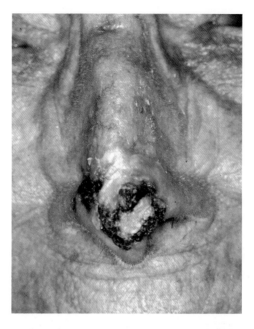

Figure 21.3 Squamous carcinoma of the skin of the nose. (Courtesy of Mr David Richardson, FRCS, Liverpool.)

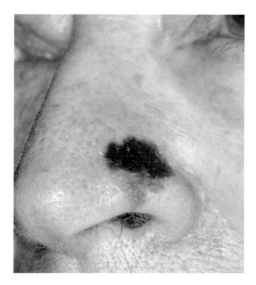

Figure 21.4 Malignant melanoma of the skin of the nose. (Courtesy of Mr David Richardson, FRCS, Liverpool.)

Treatment of facial skin cancer

- Surgery is the commonest modality. The tumour is excised with closure of the defect by primary suture if it is very small, or by the use of grafts or flaps if larger. A **graft** is a portion of tissue moved to a recipient site where it then develops its own blood supply. A **flap** is transplanted to its new site but maintains an attachment to its own blood supply. A **free flap** is a block of tissue transposed with its blood vessels which are then anastomosed to vessels at the new site. A free flap can use tissue well distant from the defect that needs to be replaced, whereas the far more commonly used local flap uses tissue from adjacent to the defect (Figs 21.5 and 21.6).

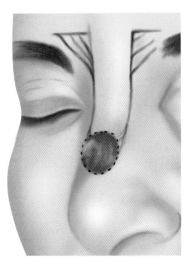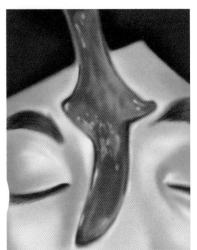

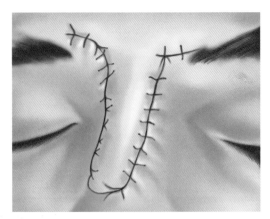

Figure 21.5 A simple advancement flap used to get a good aesthetic result following excision of a skin cancer on the dorsum of the nose.

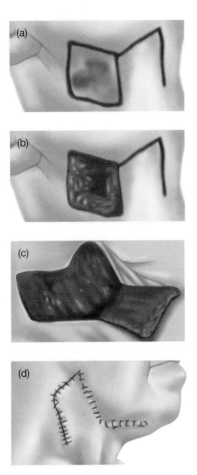

Figure 21.6 A transposition flap (in this case a 'rhomboid' flap) is used to repair the defect following excision of a skin cancer on the cheek. (a) The incision lines are marked. (b) The cancer, with a good surrounding margin, is removed. (c) The flap is developed. (d) The flap in position showing a good aesthetic result.

- **Mohs Micrographic Surgery (MMS)** is a technique involving serial histological analysis by frozen section to ensure precise removal of disease with minimal excision of normal skin and subcutaneous tissue.
- **Radiotherapy** may be needed for advanced tumours, as an adjunct to surgery or in areas of the face where reconstruction may be especially difficult.

Adequate follow-up is important, and patients are at risk of further tumours.

The treatment of cutaneous malignant melanoma can be especially challenging and require a multi-disciplinary team (MDT) approach.

Aesthetic ('cosmetic') facial surgery

Many patients seek advice because they want to change their facial appearance. Facial plastic surgeons offer an increasingly diverse range of techniques to counteract the effects of aging, injury or disease.

Blepharoplasty

This is a repair of the upper or lower eyelids and is one of the commonest techniques to restore a more youthful appearance to the ageing face.

Rhytidectomy

More commonly known as a 'facelift'

Rhinoplasty

This is surgery to alter the shape of the nose. It is often combined with nasal septal surgery – **Septorhinoplasty (SRP)** – and may be considered not just for aesthetic reasons but to improve the nasal air passages, especially there is a history of trauma. A saddle deformity of the nose can be corrected by the insertion of a graft – often a portion of the patient's cartilage – to give bulk to the dorsum of the nose – '**Augmentation Rhinoplasty**'.

Rhinophyma

This is a swollen reddened and nodular nose due to hyperplasia of the sebaceous glands. It occurs mainly in elderly men. Surgery gives good results but may need to be repeated.

Other techniques used in facial plastic surgery include fillers – typically collagen – injected into the tissues to give bulk, chemical peels or dermabrasion to remove superficial layers of skin and Botulinus toxin (Botox TM) to smooth wrinkles.

CLINICAL PRACTICE POINTS

- Prolonged exposure to sunlight is a common cause of skin cancers especially in fair-skinned people.
- Even innocent looking skin lesions on the face may be cancerous. Be vigilant and refer early.

Go to **www.lecturenoteseries.com/ENT** to test yourself using the interactive MCQs.

Part 3

The head and neck

22

Adenoids

Applied basic science

The adenoids are part of a circle of lymphoid tissue – **Waldeyer's ring** – which surrounds the entrance to the upper aerodigestive tract. Waldeyer's ring includes the palatine tonsils, lymphoid tissue in the tongue base – lingual tonsils – and a few discrete aggregates of submucosal lymphoid follicles dispersed throughout the pharynx. The adenoids are found in the nasopharynx, behind the soft palate projecting from the posterior pharyngeal wall. They occupy a large part of the space in the nasopharynx in young children. Their function is that of the pharyngeal lymphoid tissue in general, i.e. to mount an immunological response to infective agents. They are small at birth, enlarge due to hypertrophy and hyperplasia during the first 5 years of life, and regress from about the age of 7 years to adolescence, when they have all but disappeared.

In some children – mainly up to the age of 5 years – repeated upper respiratory infections cause pathological adenoidal enlargement so that the airway is obstructed. The child will mouth-breathe, snore continuously and in severe cases develop obstructive sleep apnoea (OSA) – Chapter 24. Continued mouth breathing causes drying of the throat and predisposes to chest infections. The submucosal lymphoid tissue is colonized by bacteria and may give rise to repeated upper respiratory infections, in particular rhinosinusitis and otitis media. It is thought that bacteria in the adenoids can form a protective polymeric matrix (**biofilm**) which makes penetration by antibiotics and the child's host defence mechanisms difficult. The sheer bulk of the adenoids may obstruct the opening of the Eustachian tube and contribute to middle ear disease in this way. 'Adenoidal' children may have a hyponasal quality to their speech as the normal resonance associated with a clear nasopharynx is lost, e.g. the child will pronounce *'mummy and nanny'* as *'bubby and daddy'*.

Diseases of the Ear, Nose and Throat Lecture Notes, Eleventh edition. Ray Clarke. © 2014 John Wiley & Sons Ltd.
Published 2014 by John Wiley & Sons, Ltd.

Clinical effects

Adenoids are often incorrectly blamed for a variety of childhood conditions. The main adverse effects of adenoids are:

- nasal obstruction
- pharyngitis (due to dry mouth)
- obstructive sleep apnoea (OSA)
- rhinosinusitis
- recurrent upper respiratory infections
- otitis media

Presentation and diagnosis

The history will confirm the features mentioned above. Nasal obstruction and mouth breathing are often apparent during the consultation. The adenoids are not seen during a routine examination of the nose and throat but a good view can now be had with an endoscope introduced into the nose, a procedure often surprisingly well tolerated by children (Fig. 22.1). Enlarged adenoids can also be seen by mirror examination (Fig. 22.2). A lateral soft tissue X-ray of the neck will show a shadow in the postnasal space delineating the adenoids but is now rarely needed as endoscopy is so much easier (Fig. 22.3).

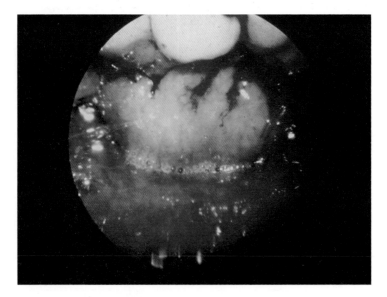

Figure 22.1 Endoscopic view of the adenoids.

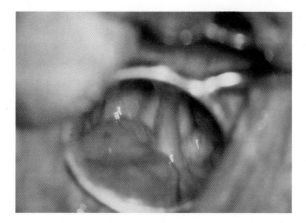

Figure 22.2 Mirror view of the nasopharynx showing adenoid tissue and the posterior end of the nasal septum (viewed under general anaesthetic).

Treatment

There are no absolute indications for adenoidectomy but it is considered for:

- Persistent rhinitis that fails to respond to medical treatment
- OSA
- Some cases of otitis media, particularly otitis media with effusion (OME, Chapter 12) that have recurred despite previous treatment with grommets. In children with recurrent ear disease, there is some evidence that 'adjuvant adenoidectomy' i.e. adenoidectomy in conjunction with grommet insertion improves outcomes in younger children.

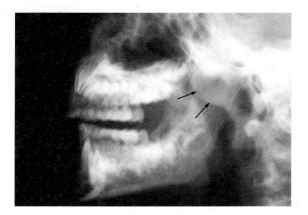

Figure 22.3 A lateral soft tissue X-ray showing adenoid enlargement.

Adenoidectomy is carried out under general anaesthesia with endotracheal intubation. An adenoid curette is swept down the posterior pharyngeal wall, taking care to remove all remnants of lymphoid tissue. Some ENT surgeons prefer to use a suction-diathermy device under direct vision to reduce bleeding.

Complications

- Haemorrhage – this usually occurs in the first 24 hours. Do not delay in setting up a drip, getting blood cross-matched and returning the child to theatre.
- Otitis media.
- Regrowth of residual adenoid tissue.
- '*Rhinolalia aperta*'. This is a disorder of speech characterized by escape of air from the nose during articulation. Removal of large adenoids in a child with a short soft palate may result in palatal incompetence. Resolution usually occurs without treatment, but if not, speech therapy is advisable.

 CLINICAL PRACTICE POINTS

- The indications for adenoidectomy are often very different to the indications for tonsillectomy.
- Assess each child for adenoidectomy on an individual basis rather than automatically suggesting 'adenotonsillectomy'.

Go to **www.lecturenoteseries.com/ENT** to test yourself using the interactive MCQs.

The oropharynx and tonsils

Applied basic science

The pharynx is the entrance to both the airway and the digestive tract. It is divided into three parts – the **nasopharynx** (postnasal space) between the skull base and the hard palate, the **oropharynx** between the hard palate and the hyoid bone, and the **hypopharynx** between the hyoid bone and the lower part of the cricoid cartilage of the larynx (Fig. 23.1).

The tonsils are in the oropharynx.

Acute and chronic pharyngitis (sore throat)

Acute pharyngitis is common and usually starts as a virus infection. It is often associated with acute rhinosinusitis as part of an upper respiratory tract infection (URTI).

The patient complains of dysphagia and malaise; on examination, the pharyngeal mucosa is hyperaemic and there may be some swelling and tenderness in the neck glands.

Chronic pharyngitis produces a persistent though mild soreness of the throat, usually with a complaint of dryness and a persistent cough as the patient tries to clear her throat.

Predisposing factors to look for are:

- tobacco use (including passive smoking and betel nut chewing);
- Chronic Obstructive Pulmonary Disease (COPD);
- mouth breathing as a result of nasal obstruction;
- rhinosinusitis;
- periodontal disease.

Treatment is symptomatic but the causes listed above may warrant treatment in their own right.

Diseases of the Ear, Nose and Throat Lecture Notes, Eleventh edition. Ray Clarke. © 2014 John Wiley & Sons Ltd.
Published 2014 by John Wiley & Sons, Ltd.

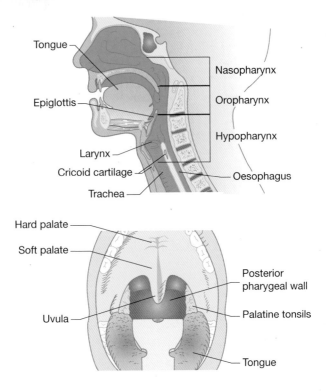

Figure 23.1 The divisions of the pharynx and oropharynx. Source: Munir and Clarke 2013. *Ear, Nose and Throat at a Glance*. With permission of John Wiley & Sons Ltd.

Treatment of acute pharynigitis

- Good analgesia. Paracetamol is usually adequate but in severe cases consider a short course of Non Steroidal Anti Inflammatory agents or Codeine.
- Plenty oral fluids. Encourage the patient to drink to prevent dehydration.
- Give antibiotics in severe cases. Simple viral sore throats do not warrant antibiotics, which are ineffective. If there is evidence of bacterial infection – e.g. pus, severe pain on swallowing or prolonged unresponsive symptoms penicillin remains the treatment of choice. If the child cannot swallow, you may need to give intravenous antibiotics.

Acute tonsillitis

Mostly occurs in children and young adults. Initial infection is typically viral but bacteria may supervene. *Streptococcus pyogenes* is still an important pathogen.

Symptoms

- Sore throat and dysphagia. Swallowing is painful. Young children may not complain of sore throat but they will be fractious and refuse to eat.
- Earache as a result of referred pain.
- Headache and malaise.

Signs

- Pyrexia may lead to febrile convulsions in susceptible infants.
- The tonsils are enlarged and hyperaemic and may exude pus.
- The pharynx is red, swollen and inflamed.
- Foetor (bad breath).
- The cervical lymph nodes are enlarged and tender.

Complications of acute tonsillitis

- Acute otitis media.
- Peritonsillar abscess (quinsy).
- Parapharyngeal abscess.
- Retropharyngeal abscess.
- Pulmonary infections (pneumonia, etc.).
- Glomerulonephritis.
- Rheumatic fever.
- Scarlet fever.

Scarlet fever is a streptococcal tonsillitis with a punctate erythematous rash, and a 'strawberry' tongue. Rheumatic fever and glomerulonephritis are due to immune complex deposition secondary to streptococcal tonsillitis. They are now rare conditions in the developed world.

Quinsy (peritonsillar abscess)

A quinsy is a collection of pus forming outside the capsule of the tonsil but within the peri-tonsillar tissue. It is more common in young adults than in children.

The patient, already suffering from acute tonsillitis becomes more ill, has a peak of temperature and develops severe dysphagia with referred otalgia. On examination, a most striking and constant feature is trismus; the buccal mucosa is often furred and there is foetor.

The quinsy pushes the tonsil downwards and medially (Fig. 23.2).

Retropharyngeal abscess

Infection can track in to the lymph nodes behind the pharyngeal wall especially in infants (Fig. 23.3). The child is obviously ill, dribbling and has a high temperature.

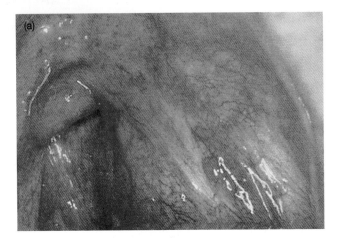

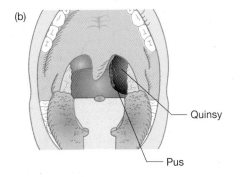

Figure 23.2 (a) and (b) Quinsy. Source (b): Munir and Clarke 2013. *Ear, Nose and Throat at a Glance*. With permission of John Wiley & Sons Ltd.

There may be airway obstruction. Inspection and palpation of the posterior pharyngeal wall reveals a smooth bulge, usually on one side of the midline.

Give intravenous antibiotics in full doses, keep the child well hydrated and refer for incision of the abscess without delay. General anaesthesia is advisable but requires a lot of skill and care as the abscess can burst with pus tracking into the airway.

Treatment of quinsy

Treatment is intravenous antibiotics and drainage of the abscess. The patient will then spit out pus and some blood, and the relief is immediate and dramatic. Drainage of quinsy is rarely needed in children, and may require general anaesthesia.

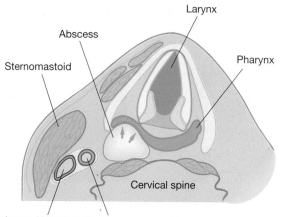

(a)

Larynx

Abscess

Sternomastoid

Pharynx

Internal jugular vein Common carotid artery

Cervical spine

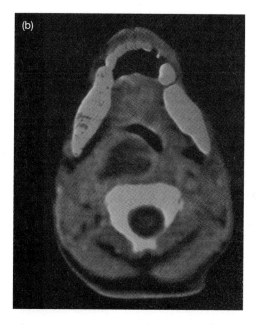

(b)

Figure 23.3 (a) Retropharyngeal abscess. Note the proximity to the larynx and to the great vessels in the parapharyngeal space. (b) CT scan showing pus.

Parapharyngeal abscess

Infection can spread beyond the pharynx and into the neck (Fig. 23.4). High-dose intravenous antibiotics and sometimes drainage will be needed.

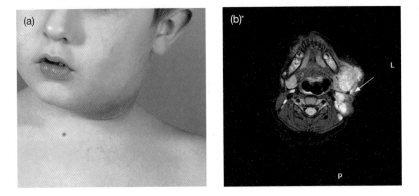

Figure 23.4 (a) Parapharyngeal abscess. (b) Scan showing parapharyngeal abscess cavity (arrowed).

Rarer forms of acute tonsillitis

Infectious mononucleosis

Infectious mononucleosis (glandular fever) usually presents as severe membranous tonsillitis. The node enlargement is marked and malaise is more severe than expected from tonsillitis (Fig. 23.5). Diagnosis is confirmed by lymphocytosis on the blood film and by the **Paul Bunnel** test. Within a week the *Monospot* blood test becomes positive. The cause is the Epstein–Barr virus and spread is by close contact. Adolescents are especially susceptible ('kissing disease').

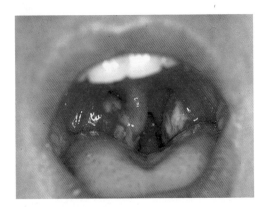

Figure 23.5 The appearance of the tonsils in glandular fever.

Diphtheria

Diphtheria is now very rare but isolated cases may still occur. Onset can be rapid and characterized by a grey membrane (difficult to remove) on the tonsils, fauces and uvula. Pyrexia is usually low and diagnosis is confirmed by examination and culture of a swab.

Agranulocytosis

Agranulocytosis is manifested by ulceration and membrane formation on the tonsils and oral mucosa. Patients on chemotherapy or with very poor immunity are especially at risk. The neutropenia is diagnostic.

HIV

Patients with impaired immunity from HIV infection are particularly at risk of pharyngitis and ulcerative tonsillitis. Opportunistic organisms including fungi can be implicated and treatment may need to be prolonged.

Tonsillectomy

Tonsillectomy rates vary greatly, not only between countries, but in different regions in the same country. Tonsillectomy is undertaken in children much more frequently than in adults (2 to 1). The operation is widely performed in well-to-do Western communities, less frequently in the developing world. Indications remain controversial, but the evidence base is improving. Common reasons for tonsillectomy are:

- Recurrent sore throats (see SIGN guidelines below).
- Obstructive sleep apnoea (OSA) (See Chapter 30).
- Suspected malignancy or lymphoma.

Treatment of recurrent acute tonsillitis

Most people will at some time experience acute tonsillitis; some are subject to recurrent attacks, especially in childhood. Between attacks the patient is usually symptom-free and the tonsils appear healthy. If such attacks are frequent and severe, tonsillectomy may be considered. The indications for tonsillectomy have changed greatly in recent years despite continuing uncertainty. Mild sore throats in children are best managed without surgery – **'watchful waiting'**. Tonsillectomy is recommended for recurrent severe sore throat in adults. The SIGN (Scottish Intercollegiate Guidance Network) guidelines – www.sign.ac/uk – are based on a review of current evidence and suggest that patients having tonsillectomy for recurrent sore throat should meet the following criteria:

- sore throats are due to acute tonsillitis (check the clinical features above);
- the episodes of sore throat are disabling and prevent normal functioning;

- seven or more well documented, clinically significant, adequately treated sore throats in the preceding year; or
- five or more such episodes in each of the preceding 2 years; or
- three or more such episodes in each of the preceding 3 years.

Post-operative care

Tonsillectomy is painful, especially in the first 10 days or so after surgery. Adequate analgesia and hydration are essential. The appearance of the tonsil beds often causes alarm. They may be covered with a white or yellowish exudate, which persists for up 2 weeks. This is quite normal and does not indicate infection. It is not pus (Fig. 23.6).

The main complication is bleeding. This can occur at or just after surgery (primary bleed, sometimes needing a second operation to control the bleeding). More often it occurs in the week or so after surgery (secondary bleed) when it is thought to be due to infection of the tonsil beds and usually improves after a few days antibiotics Fig. 23.6).

Tonsillar enlargement

Many parents are concerned about the size of their child's tonsils but no treatment is needed unless the child is subject to recurring attacks of acute tonsillitis or the tonsils are obstructing the airway (see Chapter 24). Very rarely a lymphoma presents as a unilateral tonsillar enlargement but some degree of asymmetry of the tonsils is normal in children.

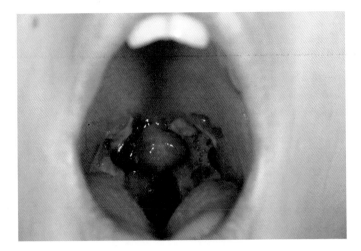

Figure 23.6 The throat one day after a tonsillectomy. This appearance is normal.

Malignant disease of the tonsil and pharynx

Carcinoma

Carcinoma will present as painful ulceration with induration of the tonsil or pharyngeal wall. There is often earache (referred pain) and slight bleeding. Lymphatic spread to the neck nodes is early. If you suspect a tonsil cancer refer the patient urgently to a head and neck clinic for assessment and a biopsy.

Lymphoma

Lymphoma of the tonsil tends not to ulcerate, but produces painless enlargement of the affected tonsil. Again, refer for an urgent biopsy if you are suspicious.

🔍 CLINICAL PRACTICE POINTS

- Most sore throats are viral, short-lived and do not require antibiotics.
- A decision to proceed to tonsillectomy should be based on good evidence, e.g. the SIGN guidelines.
- Tonsillectomy is painful. Patients need prolonged analgesia and hydration.

Go to www.lecturenoteseries.com/ENT to test yourself using the interactive MCQs.

24

Snoring and obstructive sleep apnoea syndrome (OSAS)

Snoring is the low-pitched noise brought about mainly by vibration of the pharynx. This is sometimes called 'stertorous' breathing and is a sign that there is at least some degree of airway obstruction. The noise is typically worse when the patient is asleep because the pharyngeal muscles relax and become atonic, causing narrowing or even – for brief periods – closure of the airway. The far more serious condition of obstructive sleep apnoea syndrome **(OSAS)** is characterized by episodes of **obstructive** airflow during **sleep** so that the patient stops breathing **(apnoea)** despite continuing respiratory efforts. Partial obstruction can cause greatly reduced airflow **(hypopnea)**. These episodes of apnoea can be prolonged – ten seconds or more – and cause reduced blood oxygen tension – **hypoxaemia**. The respiratory centre in the brain-stem stimulates another cycle of breathing and the patient wakes up to restore the blood oxygen. Multiple disruptions to sleep give rise to daytime tiredness. Repeated hypoxaemia can cause serious cardiovascular disease such as **hypertension, stroke, cardiac failure** and eventually **pulmonary hypertension**.

OSAS is a major public health problem, especially in wealthy Western communities where it is associated with obesity.

Snoring is a common clinical problem and is now recognized as part of a spectrum of sleep related breathing disorders (SRBD) with OSAS at the extreme end. Men are much more commonly affected.

Predisposing factors

The predisposing factors are:

- obesity, probably due to deposition of fatty tissue around the airway;
- nasal or pharyngeal obstruction e.g. rhinitis, tonsils and adenoids in children;
- increasing age;
- alcohol;
- smoking.

Adverse effects

Snoring causes a lot of marital disharmony and social isolation. Patients with OSAS may in addition suffer from:

- poor work performance;
- excessive daytime sleepiness (EDS);
- increased risk of road traffic accidents due to falling asleep;
- cardiovascular complications.

Diagnosis

Take a careful history in all patients who snore. Enquire especially about daytime sleepiness. The sleeping partner may be able to tell you if the patient stops breathing. Examine the upper respiratory tract for any evidence of obstruction and pay particular attention to the patient's weight and cardiovascular status. If there is any suspicion of OSAS refer for sleep studies, as clinical diagnosis is unreliable. These involve measuring blood oxygen tension and a variety of respiratory variables over a few hours of sleep.

Treatment of OSAS in adults

- Lifestyle modification. Try simple measures such as weight loss and avoidance of alcohol at night.
- Treat rhinitis.
- For uncomplicated snoring various devices that improve the calibre of the nasal airway or splint the jaw forward to improve the pharyngeal airway are available.
- For established OSAS, treatment with continuous pressure inspired air delivered by a face-mask or nasal prongs at night may be needed – continuous positive airway pressure - CPAP (see Fig. 24.1).
- Surgery to improve the airway is a last resort and results are uncertain

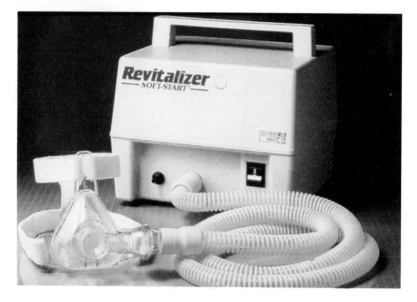

Figure 24.1 Continuous Positive Airway Pressure (CPAP) is usually administered via a facemask. An electric motor generates a constant gentle stream of air which is channelled into the delivery system. This positive pressure air column helps to splint the airway, preventing collapse of the pharyngeal walls during periods of hypotonia and overcoming obstruction

Snoring and OSAS in children

Snoring is very common in the preschool child. In otherwise healthy children, it is often associated with large tonsils and adenoids. Mild snoring on its own probably needs no treatment. OSA in children can cause not daytime sleepiness but excessive activity and behaviour problems. There is increasing evidence that it can adversely affect school performance.

Treatment of OSAS in children

* Treat rhinitis.
* If the child has evidence of persistent OSAS refer to an ENT surgeon who may recommend adenotonsillectomy.
* Snoring and OSAS in children with special needs e.g. Down syndrome or cerebral palsy, can be particularly difficult to manage and referral for multidisciplinary management is best

CLINICAL PRACTICE POINTS

- Snoring is not just a nuisance; it can be a serious medical problem.
- OSAS is underdiagnosed and undertreated.
- Treatment of OSAS in adults is mainly focussed on lifestyle changes, especially weight loss.

 Go to **www.lecturenoteseries.com/ENT** to test yourself using the interactive MCQs.

25

The larynx: applied basic science and examination

Anatomy of the larynx

The larynx or voice-box is part of the upper respiratory tract. It is lined with ciliated columnar epithelium except over the vocal folds or 'cords' which are covered with squamous epithelium. It is made of a series of cartilages, the main ones being the epiglottis, the cricoid cartilage (a complete ring just above the trachea) and the thyroid cartilage, which you can palpate as the 'Adam's Apple' externally in the neck. Various membranes, muscles and ligaments complete the structure of the larynx (Figs 25.1 and 25.2).

Physiology of the larynx

Air passes through the vocal folds, which vibrate like the reed of a musical instrument in expiration to produce voice (phonation). The other functions of the larynx are as a conduit for air entry into the respiratory tract and to close off the air-passages during swallowing to protect the lungs.

Symptoms and signs of laryngeal disease

Lesions on or around the vocal cords cause **hoarseness**.

Failure of the laryngeal inlet to close on swallowing causes **aspiration**; the patient will cough and splutter on swallowing – food 'going down the wrong way'.

Diseases of the Ear, Nose and Throat Lecture Notes, Eleventh edition. Ray Clarke. © 2014 John Wiley & Sons Ltd. Published 2014 by John Wiley & Sons, Ltd.

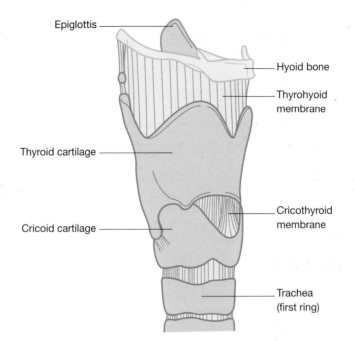

Epiglottis

Hyoid bone

Thyrohyoid membrane

Thyroid cartilage

Cricothyroid membrane

Cricoid cartilage

Trachea (first ring)

Figure 25.1 The main cartilages and membranes of the larynx.

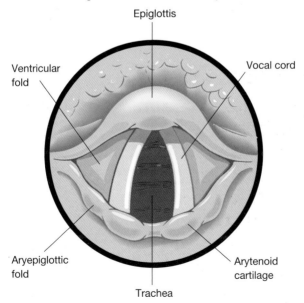

Epiglottis

Ventricular fold

Vocal cord

Aryepiglottic fold

Arytenoid cartilage

Trachea

Figure 25.2 The structures seen on indirect laryngoscopy.

The most dangerous laryngeal pathology is narrowing of the airway. This causes reduced air entry and turbulent flow so that the patient makes a high-pitched noise when breathing **(stridor).** Increasing difficulty causes a rise in respiratory rate (tachypnoea), and the patient will struggle to breathe and become distressed as he uses the accessory muscles of respiration to maintain airflow. In severe cases there may be cyanosis, cessation of air entry (apnoea) and death.

Examination of the larynx

You can get some idea of how the larynx is working by listening to the patient's **voice** (is he hoarse?) and observing his breathing (is there stridor?). Palpate the neck as well and feel for the prominence of the laryngeal cartilages. **'Crepitus'** or a sensation of 'crackling' under your fingers when you gently move the larynx is normal.

Inspecting the larynx requires some skill and practice. **Fibre-optic laryngoscopy** is increasingly available and fibre-optic instruments are now of extremely high quality. The instrument is passed through the nose into the pharynx. It is then manoeuvred past the epiglottis until the interior of the larynx is seen (Fig. 25.3). This allows inspection of the cords during phonation and also enables a photographic record to be made. To assess mobility of the cords ask the patient to say 'EE', causing adduction (movement of the cords towards the midline) or to take a deep breath, which causes abduction (movement of the cords away from the midline). The patient can even see her own larynx on a television monitor.

For **indirect laryngoscopy** ask the patient to protrude her tongue, which is held gently between the examiner's middle finger and thumb (Figs 25.4 and 25.5). A warmed laryngeal mirror is introduced gently but firmly against the soft palate in the midline. By tilting the laryngeal mirror, the various structures shown in Fig. 25.2 can be seen.

For more detailed examination and particularly if a biopsy is needed direct laryngoscopy under general anaesthesia is required (Figs 25.6 and 25.7).

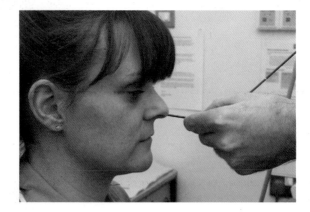

Figure 25.3 Flexible laryngoscopy.

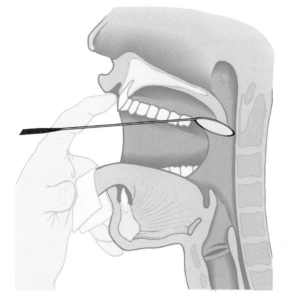

Figure 25.4 The position of the mirror on indirect laryngoscopy.

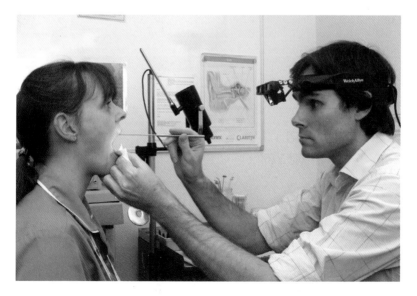

Figure 25.5 The technique of indirect laryngoscopy.

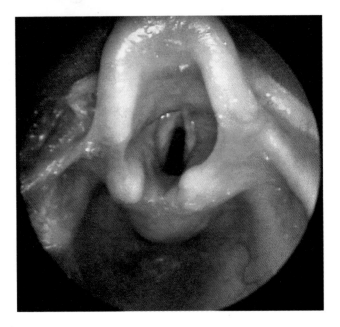

Figure 25.6 The normal larynx as seen by direct laryngoscopy in a child.

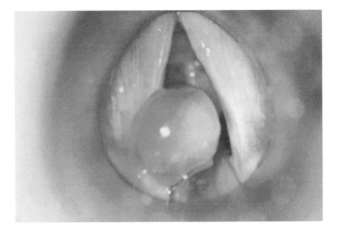

Figure 25.7 The appearance of the larynx as seen by direct laryngoscopy. Note the large polyp on the left vocal cord.

CLINICAL PRACTICE POINT

* The main symptoms and signs of laryngeal disease are hoarseness, stridor and aspiration. All are potentially serious but be especially vigilant if there is any worry about airway obstruction, which can progress very quickly.

Go to **www.lecturenoteseries.com/ENT** to test yourself using the interactive MCQs.

26

Inflammatory disorders of the larynx

Acute laryngitis: adults

Clinical features

- Aphonia (the voice is lost or reduced to a whisper).

Or

- Dysphonia (hoarseness).
- Cough – sometimes painful.
- Stridor – rare but potentially serious.

Examination by indirect laryngoscopy or using a flexible endoscope shows a red swollen larynx, sometimes with stringy mucus between the cords.

Aetiology

Acute laryngitis is more common in the winter months. It is usually caused by a virus, e.g. acute coryza (common cold).

Predisposing factors

- Upper respiratoy tract infection (URTI)
- Overuse of the voice
- Smoking (active or passive)
- Alcohol

Diseases of the Ear, Nose and Throat Lecture Notes, Eleventh edition. Ray Clarke. © 2014 John Wiley & Sons Ltd.
Published 2014 by John Wiley & Sons, Ltd.

Acute laryngotracheobronchitis or 'croup' in children

Acute laryngotracheobronchitis (ALTB) or 'croup' is very common in the winter months, especially in children under 2 years old. As a result of an acute viral upper respiratory infection, the laryngeal and tracheobronchial mucosa becomes swollen and oedematous. The child is unwell, typically with a harsh 'croupy' cough and a hoarse voice. Progressive airway obstruction can follow. The prognosis in ALTB or 'croup' is much better now that steroids are routinely used in the primary care management.

Treatment of laryngitis

- Voice rest (very difficult in practice).
- Inhalations with steam or menthol
- Avoid smoking (active and passive).
- Antibiotics are sometimes needed.

Acute epiglottitis (children)

Acute epiglottitis is a localized infection of the upper part of the larynx usually caused by *Haemophilus influenza type B (Hib)*. It causes severe swelling of the epiglottis, which obstructs the laryngeal inlet. In children it constitutes a most urgent emergency – the child may progress from being perfectly well to being dead within the space of a few hours due to airway obstruction. Fortunately, acute epiglottitis has now become very rare in the West because of the widespread use of Hib vaccine. Sporadic cases still occur and occasionally a similar clinical picture can be caused by other organisms, e.g. *Staphylococcus*. Worldwide, in areas where the Hib vaccine is not widely used, acute epiglottitis is still a major cause of acute airway obstruction in children.

Treatment of ALTB (Croup) in children

- Oral steroids: dexamethasone 0.6 mg/kg. as a single dose, repeated after eight hours if needed. This can also be given subcutaneously or intravenously.
- Nebulized ventolin, typically 1 mL of 1 in 1000 in 3 mL of saline, or nebulized adrenaline (epinephrine) 2 mL of 1 in 1000 in 2 mL normal saline
- Humidification/a steamy environment soothes the harsh cough.
- Paracetamol is a good analgesic and antipyretic.
- Some children will need hospital admission and rarely endotracheal intubation.

Clinical features

- The child is unwell, with increasing dysphagia.
- Drooling.
- A 'quack-like' cough.
- Stridor develops rapidly. The child will sit up, leaning forward to ease his airway.

Management of suspected acute epiglottitis

- Do not persist in examining the child's throat. You may cause spasm.
- Admit the child to hospital at once.
- Give intravenous antibiotics (amoxycillin).
- Most cases are now managed by endotracheal intubation.
- Some children will need tracheostomy.

Adult epiglottitis in adults ('supraglottitis')

In adults the pain is severe and is worsened on swallowing. It is slower to develop and to resolve than in children. Respiratory obstruction is less likely but hospital admission is still wise.

Laryngeal diphtheria

Laryngeal diphtheria is now rare in the Western world. The child is ill and usually presents with a membrane on the pharynx. Stridor suggests the spread of the membrane to the larynx and trachea. Hospital admission, antitoxin and general supportive measures can be life-saving. The child may need a tracheotomy.

Chronic laryngitis (Fig. 26.1)

Hoarseness is a serious sign and if it persists the larynx needs to be inspected by an ENT surgeon with a view to a biopsy.

Smoking, alcohol and habitual shouting/faulty voice production can cause chronic inflammatory changes in the laryngeal mucosa. Professional voice users e.g. teachers, actors, singers, are especially susceptible to laryngitis and may develop dysphonia due to laryngeal muscle imbalance.

The voice is hoarse and fatigues easily. There may be discomfort and a tendency to clear the throat.

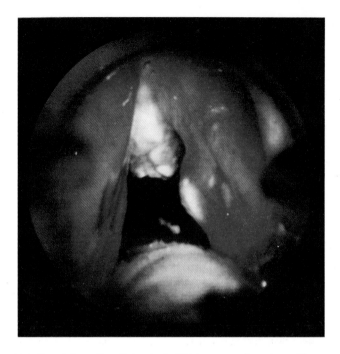

Figure 26.1 Chronic laryngitis with keratosis. This is a pre-malignant condition.

Dysplasia with disorganized mucosal cellular architecture may supervene upon chronic laryngitis. In severe cases, especially if the patient continues to smoke, this can go on to cause carcinoma.

Treatment

- The voice should be rested
- Treat upper airway sepsis
- Steam inhalations give good symptomatic relief
- Smoking is prohibited
- Voice therapy or the support of a singing teacher may be helpful

Chronic granulomatous laryngitis

Tuberculosis of the larynx is now very rare and occurs only in the presence of pulmonary tuberculosis. Treatment is by antituberculous drugs.

Syphilitic laryngitis is also extremely rare.

CLINICAL PRACTICE POINTS

- Oral steroid therapy has greatly improved the management of ALTB or 'croup' in children.
- Acute epiglottitis is now rare in the West but still potentially fatal. Admit suspected children urgently to hospital.
- Hoarseness may be a sign of serious laryngeal disease. If it persists the larynx needs to be inspected by an ENT surgeon with a view to a biopsy.

Go to www.lecturenoteseries.com/ENT to test yourself using the interactive MCQs.

Head and neck cancer

Head and neck tumours may arise from the mucosal surfaces of the aerodigestive tract – usually squamous cell carcinoma (SCC) – or from the solid organs of the head and neck, e.g. the thyroid and parathyroid glands, the salivary glands and the lymph nodes.

These tumours are far less common than lung, breast and colorectal cancers but are an important cause of morbidity and mortality especially in men. Early detection can bring about major improvements in prognosis and prompt referral is essential.

Even if non-fatal, head and neck cancer can have a devastating impact on patients' lives. Both the disease and the treatment can affect the ability to speak, swallow and breathe. Surgery can be mutilating and may require the removal of important structures such as the larynx, the tongue, parts of the pharynx and the muscles and vessels in the neck. This may necessitate replacement of surgical defects with 'flaps' including composite grafts from other parts of the body, e.g. the forearm and lower limb. Some patients will require permanent tracheostomy or laryngectomy.

The management of head and neck cancer is a subspeciality within ENT and these patients are nowadays usually looked after in designated cancer units where there is access to support facilities such as speech and language therapy, palliative care, plastic and reconstructive techniques and prostheses.

There are several histological types of head and neck cancer but Squamous Cell Carcinoma (SCC) is the commonest. The larynx, the pharynx, the oral cavity, and the nose and sinus can be the site of origin of SCC. The larynx is the site most often involved.

Aetiology

Men are more commonly affected than women. Tobacco use – including Betel nut chewing – is a major cause of SCC but Human Papilloma Virus (HPV) – is increasingly recognized as playing a key role in the development of many head and neck SCCs.

Diseases of the Ear, Nose and Throat Lecture Notes, Eleventh edition. Ray Clarke. © 2014 John Wiley & Sons Ltd.
Published 2014 by John Wiley & Sons, Ltd.

Risk factors

- Tobacco – including Betel nut chewing (causes mouth cancers, especially in South Asia (Fig. 27.1).
- Oropharyngeal HPV infection.
- Male sex.
- Older age groups.
- Lower socio-economic groups.
- Alcohol abuse.

Presentation

This depends on the site but typical clinical features are:

- hoarseness (laryngeal cancer);
- dysphagia (cancer of the pharynx);
- nonhealing ulcer – mouth and tongue cancer;
- neck mass.

Disease spread and staging

SCC spreads locally and to the regional lymph nodes in the neck (loco-regional spread). Distant metastases are rare and occur late in the disease. Cancer units

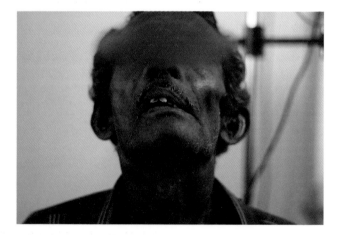

Figure 27.1 Man with neck mass and betel nut staining to teeth.

now use the TNM staging system to plan treatment and to compare results between centres. T (1–4) refers to the primary tumour, e.g. a small laryngeal tumour with no local spread is T1, an advanced tumour spread beyond the larynx is T4. N (0–3) refers to lymph nodes, N0 means no lymph node disease and N3 large nodes with advanced disease. M (0 or 1) refers to the presence (1) or absence (0) of distant metastases. A T1 N0 M0 tumour is therefore the earliest to present and the easiest to treat.

Treatment principles

One or more of three treatment modalities are usually considered for head and neck tumours:

- Radiation treatment.
- Surgery.
- Chemotherapy.

SCC is highly sensitive to radiation, hence early detection and good local control of disease by radiotherapy is the mainstay of treatment for most SCCs. Head and neck cancer patients are usually considered disease-free after 2 years as unlike many mucosal cancers distant metastases are uncommon and good loco-regional control equates to cure. Surgery may be needed for more advanced disease, for recurrence after radiotherapy or where the neck nodes are involved. In advanced disease the support of a skilled palliative care team may be invaluable. Chemotherapy has a limited role but is sometimes combined with radiation for advanced disease – **'chemoradiation'**.

SCC of the larynx

This is the commonest site for SCC in the head and neck. Cancer may develop on the vocal cords (glottic, Fig. 27.2) above the cords (supraglottic) or below (subglottic). Glottic is the commonest and typically presents early with hoarseness. This is a curable condition with a 90% 2 year survival after radiotherapy. Some units undertake limited surgery ('cordectomy') for this disease. Supraglottic tumours present later. Subglottic tumours may present with severe airway obstruction.

Some patients with SCC of the larynx will require surgery, e.g. if there is extensive neck disease, T3 or T4 disease or recurrence after radiotherapy. A total laryngectomy (Figs 27.3 and 27.4) will mean the patient will breathe permanently through a laryngeal 'stoma'. Many patients can learn to speak by using a valve which directs expired air from the trachea into the oesophagus and pharynx (Fig. 27.5). Some patients develop the ability to vibrate the oesophagus without a valve (oesophageal speech).

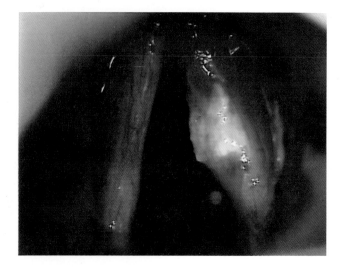

Figure 27.2 Early glottic carcinoma.

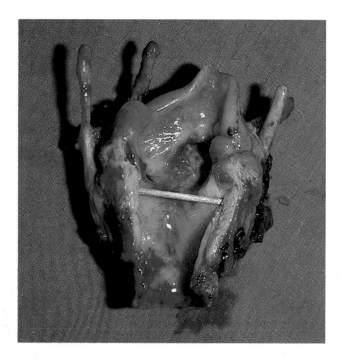

Figure 27.3 Laryngectomy specimen opened from behind, showing a left-sided carcinoma.

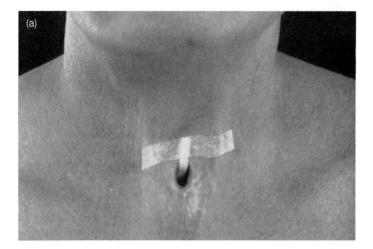

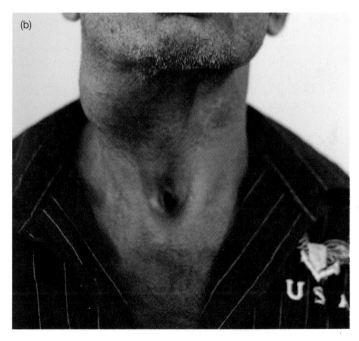

Figure 27.4 (a) A patient after total laryngectomy. (b) Recurrent disease in the neck following total laryngectomy. The patient breathes via a laryngeal stoma and has presented with a large right sided neck mass.

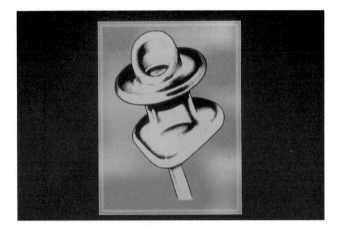

Figure 27.5 A 'Blom Singer' valve to facilitate speech after a total laryngectomy. The valve permits air to flow from the trachea to the oesophagus.

SCC of the pharynx and oral cavity

SCC of the pharynx is less common than laryngeal cancer and has a worse prognosis. Any part of the pharynx may be affected. Nasopharyngeal cancer occurs primarily in Chinese men and is considered in Chapter 25. Oropharyngeal cancer (Fig. 27.6) typically involves the tonsils (Chapter 29). The 'hypopharynx' or lower part of the pharynx, i.e. as it enters the oesophagus, is adjacent to the larynx and cancer here

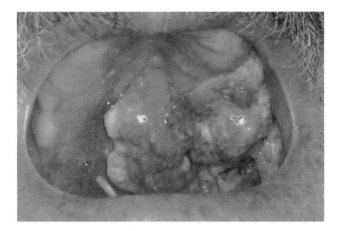

Figure 27.6 SCC of the oropharynx.

has a particularly poor prognosis. Presentation may be with dysphagia, hoarseness or both. Neck metastases are a particularly bad sign. Oral cavity tumours often present as non-healing ulcers and may be treated by excision – sometimes needing extensive flap repair – or radiotherapy depending on their extent.

🔍 CLINICAL PRACTICE POINTS

- Oropharyngeal HPV infection is now recognized as an important cause of SCC of the head and neck.
- The main presentations for head and neck cancer are hoarseness, dysphagia, a neck mass and a non-healing ulcer in the mouth or pharynx. Patients with any of these for 2 weeks or more should be considered for urgent ENT referral.
- Early detection of SCC is vital and greatly improves survival.
- Radiotherapy is the mainstay of treatment for SCC of the head and neck.

 Go to **www.lecturenoteseries.com/ENT** to test yourself using the interactive MCQs.

28

Voice disorders

The laryngeal musculature is an intricate system for varying the length, tension and degree of apposition of the vocal folds. Conditions which affect the laryngeal mucosa or the laryngeal nerves and muscles can cause changes in the voice (dysphonia) with, in severe cases, complete loss of voice (aphonia).

Voice is one of the important instruments we use to express feelings and emotions, and voice pathology can cause a great deal of psychological distress. Professional voice users such as actors, singers and teachers are especially susceptible.

The management of voice disorders (phoniatrics and phonosurgery) is now a subspeciality within ENT and many units will have a voice clinic run by an ENT surgeon and a speech and language therapist (SALT).

Symptoms of voice disorders

- Hoarseness.
- 'Rough' or 'scratchy' voice.
- 'Breathy' voice needing increased effort.
- Vocal 'fatigue' – especially after prolonged voice use.
- Changes in pitch.
- Feeling of dryness or a 'lump' in the throat.

'Muscle tension' dysphonia (MTD)

Many voice disorders are due to incoordination of the intrinsic laryngeal musculature. Symptoms vary but typically the patient will complain of having to strain to produce a good voice and that the voice tires easily. Diagnosis can be confirmed by careful endoscopic inspection of the larynx during phonation. Many voice clinics will make use of stroboscopic illumination to accentuate the subtle movements of the vocal folds. **Spasmodic dysphonia** is a variant of MTD characterized by involuntary movements of the laryngeal muscles. 'Functional' dysphonia occurs when the voice is abnormal with no apparent abnormality of laryngeal structure. Functional aphonia ('Mutism') – complete loss of voice despite an apparently normal larynx – is rare and may be due to psychological morbidity.

Factors that contribute to muscle tension dysphonia

- URTI
- Gastro-oesophageal reflux
- Smoking – active or passive
- Excessive use of the voice
- Stressful life events

Vocal cord nodules

Vocal cord nodules occur both in adults ('singer's nodules') and children ('screamer's nodules') and are thought to result from excessive vocal use. The appearance is of a small, smooth nodule on the free edge of each cord, composed of fibrous tissue covered with epithelium (Fig. 28.1). Most cases respond to voice rest and speech and language therapy (SALT). Nodules very rarely need to be removed surgically.

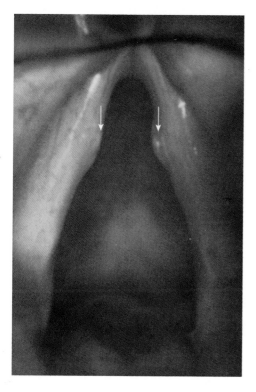

Figure 28.1 Vocal cord nodules.

Inflammatory lesions

The mucosa covering the vocal cords may become swollen and oedematous - Reinke's oedema (Fig. 28.2). Polyps, cysts, and granulation tissue may project from the free edge of the cords and interfere with normal cord apposition causing hoarseness.

Vocal cord paralysis

Usually unilateral, this presents as a hoarse breathy voice as the cords are unable to appose (Figs 28.3 and 28.4). In severe cases the patient may aspirate food and saliva as one of the functions of the cords is to close the laryngeal inlet during swallowing. The muscles responsible for moving the vocal cords are in the main supplied by the recurrent laryngeal nerves. These are branches of the vagus nerve. On the left the nerve has a longer course and winds around the aortic arch in the chest before entering the neck. Hence left recurrent laryngeal nerve palsy is more common and more likely to be caused by chest pathology. A chest X-ray is mandatory. The recurrent laryngeal nerve can be injured anywhere from the brain stem to the chest. The right or left recurrent nerve in the neck can easily be traumatized by thyroid surgery or involved in thyroid or other neck cancers.

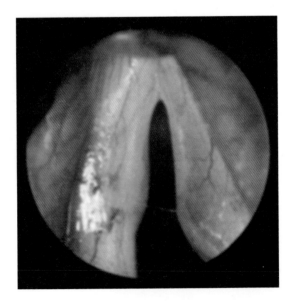

Figure 28.2 Oedematous vocal cords in Reinke's oedema, an important cause of hoarseness.

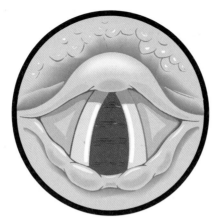

Figure 28.3 The cords in full abduction during inspiration.

Some cases of recurrent nerve palsy are idiopathic or may follow viral infections, such as influenza.

Some chest causes of left recurrent nerve palsy are:

- carcinoma of the bronchus.
- carcinoma of the oesophagus.
- malignant mediastinal nodes.
- aortic aneurysm.
- malignant neck disease
- iatrogenic (neck or chest surgery).

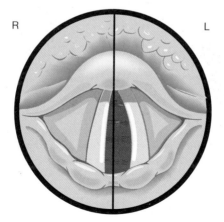

Figure 28.4 Left recurrent nerve palsy on phonation (mirror view). Note the persisting glottic aperture owing to the inability of the left cord to move to the midline.

Bilateral recurrent laryngeal nerve palsy

This occurs most commonly following surgery or malignancy of the thyroid gland, but may be the result of brain stem pathology, e.g. pseudobulbar palsy. Because the cords lie near the midline, the airway is impaired. Tracheostomy may be needed.

Treatment of voice disorders

- If there are precipitating factors such as gastro-oesophageal reflux, URTI or rhinosinusitis, these need to be treated.
- Smoking is prohibited.
- Many patients with mild MTDs need no treatment other than advice and reassurance.
- Speech and language therapy – usually focussing on specific exercises to rehabilitate the vocal muscles – is very effective.
- Interventions such as Cognitive Behaviour Therapy (CBT) may be helpful if there is psychological morbidity.
- Some voice clinics inject Botulinus toxin (Botox TM) to paralyse specific laryngeal muscles, particularly for spasmodic dysphonia.
- Surgery for voice disorders (phonosurgery) may be needed for failed conservative treatment.
- Laryngeal framework surgery includes **'thyroplasty'** operations for example to open a window in the thyroid cartilage and place silastic to move the vocal fold to the midline.
- Bulking agents such as collagen can be injected into the vocal fold to make apposition easier in vocal cord palsy.

CLINICAL PRACTICE POINTS

- Hoarseness is a serious symptom. If it persists for more than 2 weeks, refer the patient to an ENT clinic.
- Speech and language therapy (SALT) is the main treatment for voice disorders

Go to **www.lecturenoteseries.com/ENT** to test yourself using the interactive MCQs.

29

The pharynx and upper oesophagus

Applied basic science

The upper part of the pharynx (see Chapter 23) forms the start of the air passages. The lower part is continuous with the oesophagus. The swallow is described in three phases – oral, pharyngeal and oesophageal. In the pharyngeal phase, food is propelled into the oesophagus. Disorders of the pharynx and oesophagus typically present with swallowing problems.

Clinical features of pharyngo-oesophageal disorders

- **Dysphagia**. Obstruction to the passage of food causes a feeling that food won't 'go down'. If it is very severe the patient will struggle to swallow his saliva.
- **Vomiting** and reflux of food if there is severe obstruction.
- 'Odynophagia' is a painful swallow.
- 'Globus pharyngeus' is a sensation of a lump in the throat, often accompanied by discomfort on swallowing. Patients sometimes describe a 'Feeling Of Something In the Throat' (FOSIT).
- Gastro-oesophageal reflux may cause an acid taste in the mouth – 'heartburn', 'water-brash'.
- Prolonged oesophageal obstruction will cause **weight loss** and malnutrition, e.g. in oesophageal cancer.
- Beware **otalgia**. It may be referred pain from the pharynx.
- **Neck swelling** – can be due to a metastatic lymph node.

Diseases of the Ear, Nose and Throat Lecture Notes, Eleventh edition. Ray Clarke. © 2014 John Wiley & Sons Ltd. Published 2014 by John Wiley & Sons, Ltd.

Pharyngeal pouch ('hypopharyngeal diverticulum')

The pharyngeal mucosa herniates between the oblique and transverse fibres of the inferior constrictor muscle to produce a persistent pouch (Fig. 29.1). The condition occurs mostly in the elderly and is thought to be due to failure of the cricopharyngeus part of the inferior constrictor to relax during swallowing, thus building up pressure above it.

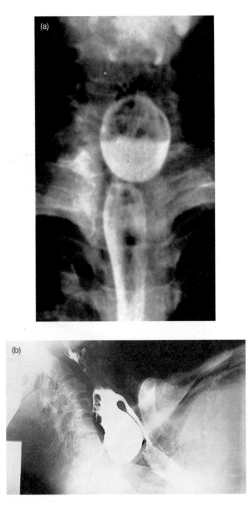

Figure 29.1 A barium swallow X-ray showing a pharyngeal pouch (a) and lateral view (b).

Clinical features

- Discomfort in the throat.
- Dysphagia as the pouch enlarges.
- Regurgitation of undigested food.
- Aspiration pneumonia.
- If the pouch is large, gurgling noises in the throat on swallowing.
- A pouch almost never causes a palpable neck swelling.

Investigation

The pouch is easily demonstrated on barium swallow (Fig. 29.1).

Treatment

An established pouch causing symptoms will require surgical treatment. Under general anaesthesia, a dilating rigid pharyngoscope is used to demonstrate the party wall between the oesophagus anteriorly and the pouch posteriorly. A staple gun is then used to divide the wall and at the same time staple the cut edges (Fig. 29.2). The patient is usually able to eat the following day and the hospital stay is very short.

It is now rarely necessary to excise a pouch by external approach through the neck.

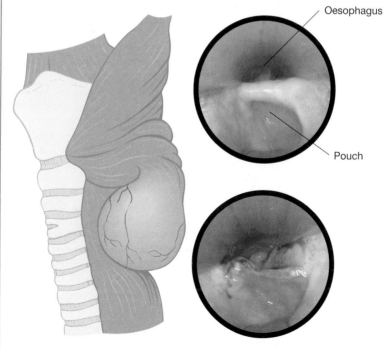

Oesophagus

Pouch

Figure 29.2 External and endoscopic views of the pharyngeal pouch. The photographs show appearances before and after endoscopic diverticulotomy with a stapling device.

Globus pharyngeus

The sensation of a 'lump in the throat' is familiar to everyone and occurs during periods of heightened emotion. It is probably due to tightening of the cricopharyngeus muscle which separates the pharynx from the oesophagus. Many patients complain bitterly of a sensation of a 'lump' or discomfort in the throat, sometimes intermittent and sometimes constant. Globus pharyngeus is the term applied to this sensation. The discomfort is often relieved by eating. There is no interference with swallowing of food or liquids.

Symptoms tend to be aggravated by the patient's constant action of swallowing, and the symptoms can cause a great deal of anxiety. A proportion of patients with globus pharyngeus have excessive reflux of gastric contents into the oesophagus and pharynx – gastro-oesophageal reflux disease **(GORD)**. Whether this association is causal or not is debated. Many patients worry that they have developed throat cancer and if symptoms persist thorough endoscopy is essential. Globus pharyngeus is one of the commonest reasons for referral to a head and neck cancer screening clinic. Older textbooks describe this condition as 'globus hystericus' reflecting its alleged psychological aetiology and its increased prevalence in women but most patients have no demonstrable psychological morbidity. Men are frequently affected.

Treatment of globus pharyngeus

- Most patients improve with reassurance reinforced by adequate examination and investigation but for many this is a troublesome and recalcitrant condition.
- Gastro-oesophageal reflux may need to be treated, e.g. with antacids, proton-pump inhibitors.

Oesophageal disorders

True dysphagia warrants immediate referral and endoscopy under the supervision of a gastro-enterologist. Oesophageal cancer is primarily a disease of the middle-aged and elderly, with a poor prognosis but with a much better outcome if detected early (Fig. 29.3) Dysphagia may also be caused by oesophageal motility disorders. This is a group of disorders – including **oesophageal spasm** and **achalasia** – characterized by abnormal patterns of movement and disordered peristalsis in the oesophagus.

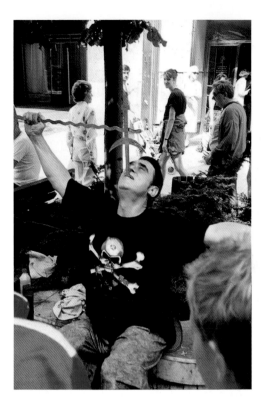

Figure 29.3 A sword swallower in Prague. The first ever oesophagoscopy was performed in the 19th century on a sword swallower by Küssmaul to demonstrate its feasibility.

> ### CLINICAL PRACTICE POINTS
> - Dysphagia is a serious symptom. Refer for urgent investigations
> - Globus pharyngeus is now the commonest reason for referral to an adult ENT clinic. Most patients respond to reassurance.

 Go to **www.lecturenoteseries.com/ENT** to test yourself using the interactive MCQs.

30

Tracheostomy

✓ Tracheotomy, the making of an opening into the trachea, is one of the oldest operations in surgery. It can be life-saving. If the operation involves the creation of a stoma - i.e. a connection between the tracheal edges and the skin - this is a tracheostomy.

Indications for tracheostomy

- To bypass upper airway obstruction.
- To protect the tracheobronchial tree.
- To facilitate artificial ventilation.

Airway obstruction

If a patient has an acutely obstructed airway and you cannot introduce an endotracheal tube, you may be able to bypass a partially obstructed airway using a 'bag and mask' (Fig. 30.1). If the patient is still not getting enough air into the

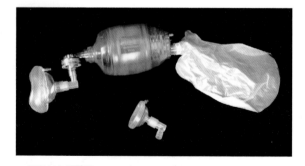

Figure 30.1 Bag and mask.

Diseases of the Ear, Nose and Throat Lecture Notes, Eleventh edition. Ray Clarke. © 2014 John Wiley & Sons Ltd. Published 2014 by John Wiley & Sons, Ltd.

lungs, tracheotomy must be done without delay. You can buy a little time until more experienced help is available by inserting a wide-bore needle into the cricothyroid membrane (Fig. 30.2). Most tracheotomies nowadays are done in more controlled conditions, under general anaesthesia and with an endotracheal tube in place.

Some causes of upper airway obstruction

- Congenital
  - Subglottic or upper tracheal stenosis.
  - Laryngeal web.
- Trauma
  - Prolonged endotracheal intubation.
  - Neck injuries, gunshot wounds and cut throat, laryngeal fracture.
- Infections
  - Acute epiglottitis (see Chapter 26).
  - Laryngotracheobronchitis.
  - Diphtheria.
  - Ludwig's angina.
- Malignant tumours
- Bilateral vocal cord paralysis

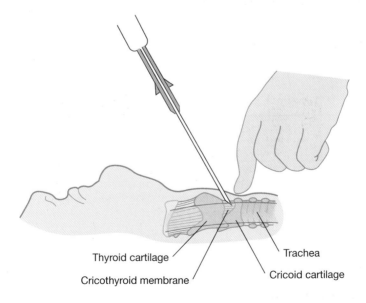

Thyroid cartilage

Cricothyroid membrane

Trachea

Cricoid cartilage

Figure 30.2 Cricothyroidotomy.

Protection of the tracheobronchial tube

Any condition causing pharyngeal or laryngeal incompetence may allow aspiration of food, saliva, blood or gastric contents. If the condition is of short duration, e.g. general anaesthesia, endotracheal intubation is best, but for chronic conditions tracheotomy may be needed. This allows easy access to the trachea and bronchi for regular suction and permits the use of a cuffed tube, which further protects against aspiration. Examples of such conditions are:

- Neurological disorders, e.g. polyneuritis (e.g. Guillain–Barré syndrome), brain stem stroke.
- Coma (if it is likely to be prolonged) e.g. due to:
  - Generalized sepsis
  - head injury
  - severe burns
  - poisoning
  - stroke

To facilitate artificial ventilation

If ventilation is to be for a long period, tracheotomy is better than an endotracheal tube. It is a lot more comfortable for the patient. Other advantages are:

- Bypass of laryngeal resistance – makes ventilation easier with lower pressures.
- Easier access to the trachea for the removal of bronchial secretions (suction).
- Easier administration of humidified oxygen.
- Positive-pressure ventilation is easier.
- 'Dead space' is reduced.

Elective tracheotomy

Surgical

Open surgical tracheotomy is best done under general anaesthesia with endotracheal intubation. Extend the neck and straighten the head . Make a transverse incision midway between the cricoid cartilage and sternal notch (Fig. 30.3). Identify and retract the strap muscles laterally (Fig. 30.4) and divide the thyroid isthmus. Find the cricoid and count the tracheal rings. Make a vertical opening into the trachea, centred on the third and fourth rings (Fig. 30.5). A single slit in the tracheal wall is best, after first inserting stay sutures on either side to allow traction on the opening in order to insert the tube.

After insertion of the tracheostomy tube, the trachea is aspirated thoroughly.

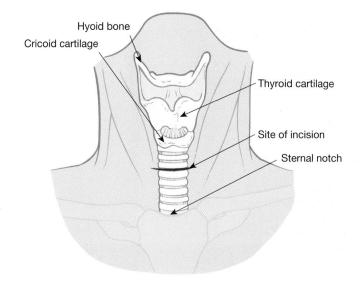

Figure 30.3 Tracheostomy showing the landmarks of the neck and the incision for operation.

Per-cutaneous tracheotomy (PCT)

Many intensive care units now recommend a percutaneous technique with a minimal skin incision, introducing a series of cannulas of increasing calibre to dilate the tracheotomy before putting in a tracheotomy tube (Fig. 30.6).

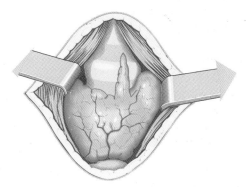

Figure 30.4 The strap muscles are retracted, exposing the trachea and the thyroid isthmus.

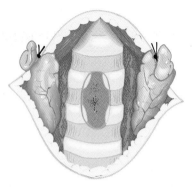

Figure 30.5 The thyroid isthmus has been divided and an opening made in the anterior tracheal wall.

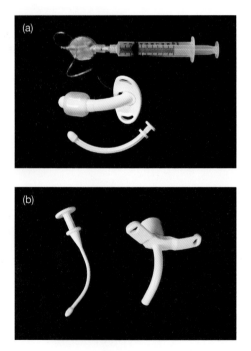

Figure 30.6 Tracheotomy tubes. (a) is an adult cuffed tracheotomy tube. The cuff can be inflated to protect the trachea and lungs from secretions and to minimize leakage. (b) is a child's tracheotomy tube with its introducer. In a small child a cuff takes up too much space and is rarely used. There is no inner tube for changing in the event of it getting blocked as the child's airway is too narrow and the inner tube would take up too much space. If the tube blocks, either clean it out immediately with suction or remove it.

After-care of the tracheotomy

Nursing care

Nursing care must be of the highest standard to keep the tube patent and prevent dislodgement.

Position

Adult patients in the post-operative period should usually be sitting well propped up; take care in infants that the chin does not occlude the tracheotomy; extend the baby's neck slightly over a soft pillow or a rolled-up towel.

Suction

Apply suction at regular intervals dictated by the amount of secretions. A clean catheter must be gently passed down into the tube in conscious patients. Unconscious or ventilated patients may also need physiotherapy.

Humidification

Humidification of the inspired air is essential to prevent drying and the formation of crusts. If necessary, sterile saline (1 mL) can be introduced into the trachea, followed by suction.

Tube changing

Tube changing should be avoided if possible for 2 or 3 days, after which the track should be well established and the tube can be changed easily. Cuffed tubes need particular attention, with regular deflation of the cuff to prevent pressure necrosis. The amount of air in the cuff should be the minimum required to prevent an air leak.

Decannulation

Decannulation should only be carried out when it is obvious that the tracheotomy is no longer required. The patient should be able to manage with the tube occluded for at least 24 h before it is removed (Fig. 30.7).

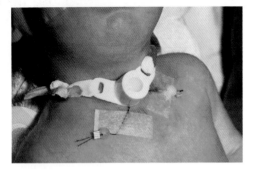

Figure 30.7 A newly performed tracheostomy in a small child. Note the stay sutures on either side to aid replacement of the tube should it become dislodged.

Complications

- Bleeding.
- Pneumothorax. Due to perforation of the pleura. This usually heals but may make post-operative care very difficult. Mediastinal emphysema can also occur.
- Obstruction of the tube or trachea by crusts of inspissated secretion may be fatal. Act quickly, remove the whole tube and replace it if blocked. If the tube is patent, explore the trachea with angled forceps to remove the obstruction. An explosive cough may expel the crust and the tube can then be replaced.
- Complete dislodgement of the tube if it is not adequately fixed. Hold the wound edges apart with a tracheal dilator and put in a clean tube. Good light is essential.
- Partial dislodgement of the tube is more difficult to recognize and may be fatal. The tube comes to lie in front of the trachea, the airway will be impaired and, if left, erosion of the innominate artery may result in catastrophic haemorrhage. Make sure that at all times the patient breathes freely through the tube.
- Surgical emphysema may occur if the patient is on positive-pressure ventilation. It is usually self-limiting.
- Perichondritis and subglottic stenosis especially if the cricoid cartilage is injured. Go below the first ring.

CLINICAL PRACTICE POINTS

- In respiratory obstruction or respiratory failure if there is no steady improvement, support the airway by endotracheal intubation or tracheotomy.
- Learn the technique of emergency tracheotomy/cricothyroidotomy.

Go to **www.lecturenoteseries.com/ENT** to test yourself using the interactive MCQs.

31

Diseases of the salivary glands

Applied basic science

The salivary glands consist of:
- The parotid glands.
- The submandibular glands.
- Minor salivary glands throughout the mouth and upper air passages. (The sublingual collection is included in this group.)

Parotid gland

The parotid gland lies on the side of the neck and face in close relationship to the ear, the angle of the mandible and the muscles of the neck. The facial nerve enters the posterior part of the parotid gland and divides within its substance into its various branches, which exit at the anterior margin of the gland. It is the presence of the facial nerve within the parotid that makes surgery of this gland so difficult. Its duct opens opposite the second upper molar tooth, where it forms a small visible papilla. Its secretomotor nerve supply comes from the glossopharyngeal nerve via the tympanic plexus in the middle ear.

The saliva produced is entirely serous. The surface outline of the gland is shown in Fig. 31.1.

The submandibular salivary gland

The submandibular gland lies in the floor of the mouth below and medial to the mandible. It is mostly below the mylohyoid muscle which forms the floor of the mouth. The deep part of the gland curves around the back of the mylohyoid and the duct runs forward to open at the sublingual papilla, one on either side of the midline. The deep part of the gland lies on the lingual nerve, from which it

Diseases of the Ear, Nose and Throat Lecture Notes, Eleventh edition. Ray Clarke. © 2014 John Wiley & Sons Ltd. Published 2014 by John Wiley & Sons, Ltd.

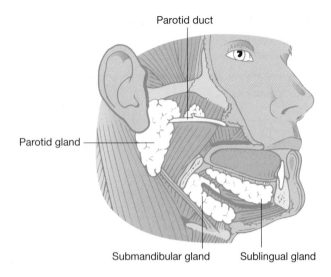

Parotid duct

Parotid gland

Submandibular gland   Sublingual gland

Figure 31.1 The surface outline of the parotid and submandibular glands. The parotid gland is larger than is usually appreciated.

receives its secretomotor supply derived from the facial nerve via the chorda tympani in the middle ear. The saliva from the submandibular gland is both serous and mucous.

The minor salivary glands

The parotid and submandibular glands are the *major* salivary glands. The *minor* salivary glands can be seen and felt in the lips, cheeks, palate and upper air passages. They produce mainly mucous saliva and are responsible for a large proportion of the total saliva secreted. They are subject to many of the diseases that affect the major salivary glands.

History-taking

- Enquire about pain and swelling of the glands in relation to eating. If the duct is obstructed, the whole gland will become tense and painful and enlarge visibly during saliva production, and will reduce slowly over about an hour.
- If there is a lump, ask about variation in size and whether it is related to food. Tumours do not enlarge during salivation, but do tend to get bigger with time.
- Ask about dryness of the mouth, remembering that obstruction of even two major glands produces little apparent change. Persistent dryness suggests diffuse salivary gland disease.
- Ask about recent contact with mumps.
- Some systemic diseases – e.g. collagen vascular diseases – can cause diffuse inflammation (sialadenitis) of the salivary glands.

Examination of the salivary glands

- Inspect the salivary glands externally, noting any swellings or asymmetry. Test the function of the facial nerve in all its divisions.
- Inspect the parotid and submandibular ducts to assess saliva flow, redness and the presence of pus or an obvious stone. Inspect the mouth to see if it is excessively dry.
- Palpate the glands. In the case of the submandibular gland put one gloved finger into the mouth as you feel the gland externally (bimanual palpation). Feel for calculi especially at the duct orifices.
- If the patient is given a sweet to suck any enlargement on salivation can be assessed.
- Check the ears.
- Examine the rest of the neck for lymph nodes.

Investigation

- Plain X-ray may show a radio-opaque calculus.
- Ultrasonic scanning is quick, non-invasive and safe. Good for masses and cysts.
- CT/MRI. If there is a large parotid tumour an MR scan will outline it well.
- Sialography. Contrast medium injected into the gland after cannulation of the duct. Invasive, less often used nowadays, but can sometimes help to flush debris from the gland.
- Sialendoscopy. Very fine endoscopes are now available to permit direct cannulation and inspection of the salivary ducts.

Inflammation of the salivary glands (sialadenitis)

Mumps

Mumps is the commonest acute inflammatory condition of salivary glands. Infection is with the mumps virus. It affects mainly the parotid glands, which become swollen and painful, but the submandibular glands may also be involved. Its incidence had fallen to very low levels as a result of immunization, but outbreaks still occur especially among teenagers and young adults who were not vaccinated. Mumps parotitis is self-limiting but complications can include deafness, orchitis with the risk of infertility in boys, and encephalitis.

Acute suppurative parotitis

This is uncommon and usually occurs in debilitated patients. Newborn babies, the elderly, malnourished patients and those with severely compromised immunity are at risk. Treatment is with antibiotics, rehydration and oral hygiene. An abscess may need surgical incision.

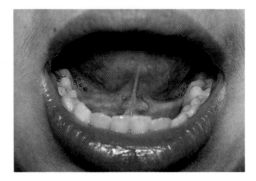

Figure 31.2 Calculus in left submandibular duct orifice.

Acute sialadenitis

Acute sialadenitis may affect the submandibular gland (commonly) or the parotid gland (rarely). Infection tracks back from the oral cavity and may be due to a stone in the duct. The patient is usually unwell with a fever. The affected gland is painful and swollen and is made worse by eating. Removal of the stone provides dramatic relief in most cases.

Salivary calculi

Most salivary calculi occur in the submandibular gland because of the mucoid nature of its saliva, which can become inspissated (Fig. 31.2). However, calculi do also occur in the parotid gland.

The flow of saliva from the affected gland becomes obstructed, causing the gland to swell during salivation. Swelling is painful and its size may be alarming. The swelling will usually resolve over about an hour.

The calculus can be seen if it presents at the duct opening, or felt within the duct or gland.

Recurrent acute inflammation

Recurrent acute inflammation of the major salivary glands typically occur in older children and adolescents and will usually subside by puberty. Treat conservatively.

Chronic inflammation

Chronic inflammation of the parotid or submandibular gland is usually due to sialectasis (duct dilatation leading to stasis and infection). The gland is thickened with episodic pain and infection, and can be felt easily on bimanual examination.

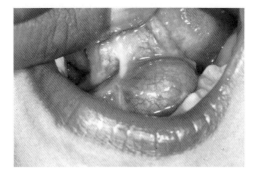

Figure 31.3 Sublingual retention cyst.

Salivary retention cysts

Salivary cysts occur most commonly in the floor of the mouth, where they may become very large and expand the loose tissues (Fig. 31.3). The name 'ranula' is often applied. Less commonly, such retention cysts occur on the mucosal aspect of the lips. They are best removed surgically.

Sjögren's syndrome

Sjögren's syndrome is an auto-immune systemic disorder affecting the salivary and lacrimal glands. There is enlargement of the glands and loss of secretion, leading to dryness of the eyes and mouth.

Treatment of sialadenitis

- Analgesia.
- Oral fluids.
- Antibiotics if there is sepsis.
- An abscess may need surgical incision and drainage.
- A submandibular duct stone may need surgical removal, but treat the infection first.
- If there is excessive dryness of the mouth, symptomatic relief can be obtained by the use of artificial saliva or glycerine and warm-water mouthwash.
- Chronic infection may cause permanent damage to the ducts and the glandular tissue (sialectesis) and if symptoms are persistent, excision of all or part of the gland may be needed. The submandibular gland so affected can be easily excised; chronic sialectasis of the parotid poses a difficult problem. Excision has a high risk of facial nerve damage and long-term antibiotics should be tried before resorting to parotidectomy (Fig. 31.4).

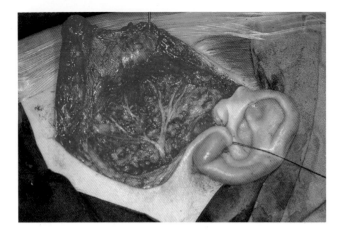

Figure 31.4 The facial nerve after superficial parotidectomy for a benign tumour in a boy aged 12 years.

Salivary gland tumours

Salivary glands contain lymph nodes within their structure and may be the site of metastases from a non-salivary primary site or from blood disorders such as leukaemia (Fig. 31.5). Lymphoma may develop in the salivary lymphoid tissue. Primary tumours of the salivary glands usually present with painless swelling of the gland.

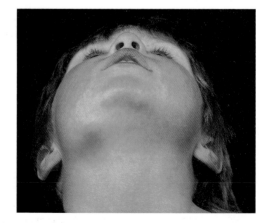

Figure 31.5 Enlarged right submandibular gland from chronic infection.

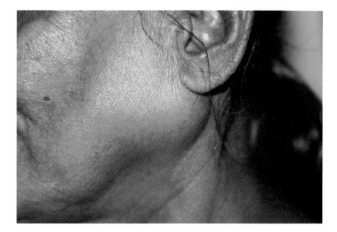

Figure 31.6 A pleomorphic adenoma in the parotid gland.

Benign tumours

- Pleomorphic salivary adenoma (mixed salivary tumour, PSA) (Fig. 31.6). By far the commonest. PSA accounts for about 90% of parotid tumours in adults. May become malignant, but tends to be slow growing. Treatment is surgical. Most frequently in the parotid gland.
- Warthin's tumour (cystic lymphoepithelial lesion).
- Haemangioma.
- Lymphoma.

Malignant tumours

- Adenoid cystic carcinoma. The commonest malignant tumour of salivary glands. With early perineural invasion, the long-term prognosis is poor but survival for many years is usual.
- Muco-epidermoid tumours.
- Acinic cell tumours.
- Malignant pleomorphic adenoma.
- Squamous carcinoma.
- Malignant lymphoma.

Drooling

While not due to disease of the salivary glands, children or adults with for example cerebral palsy or stroke may be unable to control the saliva produced, particularly from the sublingual and submandibular ducts. This causes much distress and discomfort to patient and relatives. Salivary overflow (sialorhoea) can cause eczema of the skin and soiling of the clothes. Salivary flow can be reduced by the use of hyoscine patches. Some centres advise injection of botulinus toxin (Botox TM) to the glands to paralyse secreto-motor fibres and reduce salivary flow. Some patients can also be helped by surgical relocation of the submandibular ducts to divert salivary flow. The ducts are repositioned near the tonsil and the sublingual glands are excised.

CLINICAL PRACTICE POINTS

- If a submandibular gland swelling gets bigger on eating, think of a stone in the submandibular duct.
- Parotid gland surgery is made particularly challenging because the facial nerve runs through the gland. All patients having parotidectomy must be warned of the risk of facial nerve damage.

Go to **www.lecturenoteseries.com/ENT** to test yourself using the interactive MCQs.

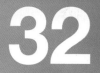

Neck lumps

A 'lump in the neck' is a common clinical scenario. It is important to have a structured approach to diagnosis and management and to know which neck lumps need urgent referral.

Any of the normal anatomical structures in the neck can become enlarged to cause a 'lump' (Fig. 32.1). In practice most neck masses are derived from the lymph nodes of the neck (cervical **adenopathy**), the thyroid gland **(goitre)** or the **salivary glands** (Chapter 39).

The range of pathologies is very different in adults and children.

Lymph nodes

Acute cervical adenopathy

Enlarged tender neck nodes are an expected feature of acute infections in the pharynx or the oral cavity, e.g. acute tonsillitis, infectious mononucleosis. In acute bacterial infection there may be suppuration in the nodes of the neck to form a painful abscess (Fig. 32.2).

Treatment of acute cervical adenopathy

- Treat the cause e.g acute tonsillitis
- Hydration – plenty oral fluids
- Analgesia
- Antibiotics for bacterial infection
- Abscess may need surgical drainage

Persistently enlarged lymph nodes

Children inevitably develop enlarged neck nodes during the course of an upper respiratory infection and as a response to various viral conditions. These enlarged nodes are often multiple and may persist for many months after the infection has subsided. Provided the nodes are of firm uniform consistency, are mobile and non-tender, and have shown no tendency to rapid change or a sudden growth spurt

Diseases of the Ear, Nose and Throat Lecture Notes, Eleventh edition. Ray Clarke. © 2014 John Wiley & Sons Ltd.
Published 2014 by John Wiley & Sons, Ltd.

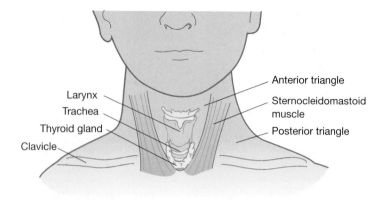

Figure 32.1 The anatomy of the neck showing its division into triangles by the sternocleidomastoid muscle. The midline structures (larynx, trachea, pharynx, oesophagus and thyroid gland) and the main vessels are in the anterior triangle. The posterior triangle contains nerves, vessels, lymph nodes and muscles.

parents can be reassured and the child can be watched. Tuberculosis is now uncommon, but should be considered in the case of large persistent nodes (Fig. 32.3).

Indications for referral

- Solitary node (exclude lymphoma).
- Sudden increase in size of nodes.

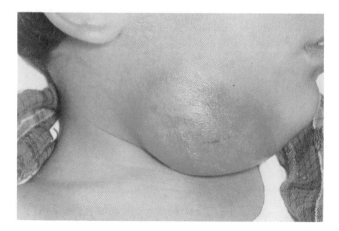

Figure 32.2 A neck abscess.

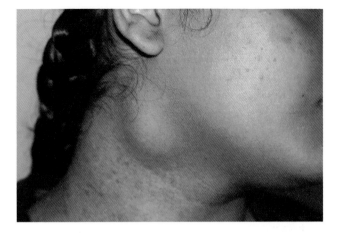

Figure 32.3 Tuberculous neck node.

- Hard rubbery nodes.
- Skin changes in the neck. Parental anxiety.
- History suggestive of systemic disease, e.g. HIV infection.

Enlarged neck nodes in adults are much more ominous. Head and neck cancer often presents in this way. If there is a clear history of acute infection then treatment with antibiotics is appropriate but a neck node that remains enlarged after 2 weeks needs urgent referral (Fig. 32.4).

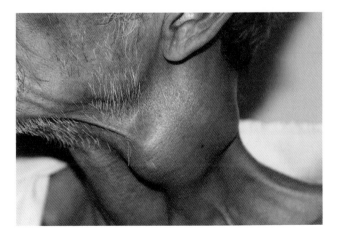

Figure 32.4 A large malignant neck node.

Investigations

Most patients with a neck node will now be seen in a rapid access head and neck clinic.

- Endoscopy of the upper aerodigestive tract may reveal a primary cancer.
- Aspiration biopsy cytology (ABC) or fine needle aspiration (FNA) can often confirm a diagnosis at a single clinic visit.
- Ultrasound can help show if a lesion is single or solitary, cystic or solid, and whether the normal architecture of the node is disrupted as in a lymphoma (Fig. 32.5).
- CT and MRI may be needed to delineate the size of a mass and plan treatment.

Some important causes of an enlarged neck node are shown in Box 32.1.

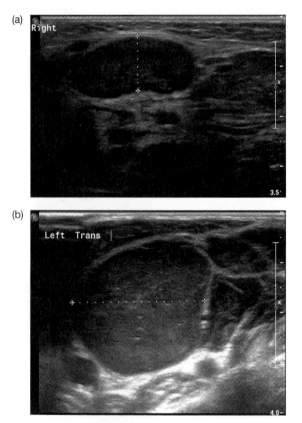

(a)

(b)

Figure 32.5 Ultrasound scanning can be an effective non-invasive aid to diagnosis. Scan (a) shows a normal neck node. Scan (b) is from a patient with a lymphoma. The normal hilar architecture is destroyed. Scanning can also be used to help ultrasound-guided FNA (fine needle aspiration) Biopsy giving an almost immediate cytological diagnosis in some conditions.

Box 32.1 Causes of an enlarged neck node

- Malignant disease
- Lymphoma
- Acute infection.
- Branchial cyst – a cystic swelling usually in young adults thought to be due to epithelial inclusions in lymph nodes.
- Chronic infection, e.g tuberculosis.
- HIV.
- A variety of chronic inflammatory diseases that cause lymphadenopathy – sometimes called **'pseudolymphoma'** and including Rosai Dorfman disease, Kikuchi's disease.

Thyroid gland swellings (goitre)

The thyroid gland is situated in the midline of the neck. Two lobes are joined by an isthmus which encircles the trachea (Fig. 32.1). An enlarged thyroid characteristically moves on swallowing (Fig. 32.6). Enlargement can be diffuse, i.e. involving the whole gland or 'nodular'. A nodular goitre may be 'multinodular' or there may be a single focus of swelling in the gland – the more worrying solitary thyroid nodule. The patient may have features of **hyperthyroidism**, **hypothyroidism** or more commonly have normal thyroid function (**'euthyroid'**).

Some important causes of thyroid swelling are shown in Box 32.2.

Box 32.2 Common thyroid swellings

- Cysts.
- Nodules, solitary or multiple, e.g. due to iodine deficiency, reactive hyperplasia.
- Inflammatory, e.g. thyroiditis.
- Benign neoplasms, e.g.adenoma.
- Malignant disease, e.g.carcinoma.

Investigation

A patient with a thyroid swelling should be referred to a head and neck/thyroid clinic. Investigations include thyroid function tests, ultrasound to determine if a nodule is cystic or solid and whether it is single or multiple, and FNA as already described for cervical lymphadenopathy. Technetium scanning (Fig. 32.7) and CT or MRI may be needed.

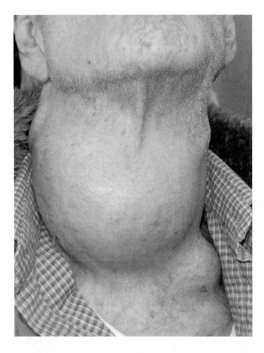

Figure 32.6 Patient with a large goitre. Courtesy of Mr S.R. Jackson, FRCS.

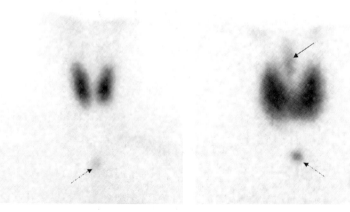

Figure 32.7 Technitium scan showing uptake in the lobes of the thyroid gland. The arrows show a marker at the sternum for orientation and the 'pyramidal lobe' of the thyroid.

Treatment of thyroid swellings

This will depend on the precise pathology. Not all goitres need treatment.

- Abnormalities of thyroid gland function may need to be managed with thyroxine or anti-thyroid drugs under the supervision of an endocrinologist.
- Radioactive iodine under the supervision of a specialist in nuclear medicine is frequently used to destroy overactive thyroid tissue.
- Most thyroid cancers are associated with a good prognosis if treated early. This will usually require surgery – partial or total thyroidectomy. Radioactive iodine may be needed to destroy residual thyroid tissue. Some patients will need thyroxine replacement therapy for life.

Thyroglossal cyst

Goitre is uncommon in children but they not infrequently present with a midline cystic neck swelling (Fig. 32.8) which moves on swallowing and on protrusion of the tongue. This is a cystic remnant of the thyroglossal duct which contributes to the descent of the thyroid gland in the embryo. It may become infected, red and painful. The treatment is surgical excision.

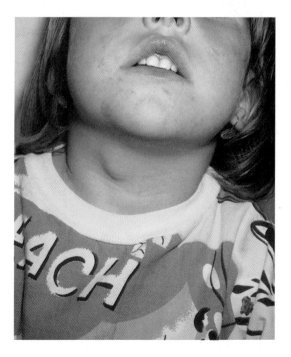

Figure 32.8 Thyroglossal cyst.

CLINICAL PRACTICE POINT

- An enlarged neck node in an adult is ominous. Refer urgently to a head and neck clinic.

Go to **www.lecturenoteseries.com/ENT** to test yourself using the interactive MCQs.

Part 4

ENT emergencies

33

Injuries of the ear and temporal bone

The pinna and external ear

Penetrating injuries

The external ear is frequently injured due to its exposed position on the side of the head. Lacerations may be due to penetrating trauma including stab wounds and bites. Clean the tissues and carefully repair them including the cartilage to get a good aesthetic result. A tear in the ear canal can be due to hairpins, clips, and cotton buds as a result of vigorous attempts to clean the ear. This can predispose to otitis externa and to stenosis of the canal. Foreign bodies in the ear canal are common, especially in children and are discussed in Chapter 6.

Very rarely, all or a part of the pinna can be avulsed. If the avulsed part is preserved and quickly reattached surgically, survival of the tissues may be possible.

Blunt injuries (haematoma auris)

Haematoma of the pinna usually occurs as a result of a shearing blow (Fig. 5.6). It is a common rugby injury, but can be due to a punch or a blow with a blunt object. The pinna is ballooned and the outline of the cartilage is lost. A layer of blood forms under the skin and subcutaneous tissues and can cause pressure necrosis if not relieved– a 'cauliflower' ear. Evacuate the clot and the reappose the layers by pressure dressings or vacuum drain.

The eardrum

The tympanic membrane is well protected. Traumatic damage when it does occur may be direct or indirect.

Diseases of the Ear, Nose and Throat Lecture Notes, Eleventh edition. Ray Clarke. © 2014 John Wiley & Sons Ltd.
Published 2014 by John Wiley & Sons, Ltd.

Direct trauma can be caused by poking in the ear with sharp implements such as hair-grips, in an attempt to clean the ear; syringing or unskilled attempts to remove wax or foreign bodies may also be to blame.

Indirect trauma is usually caused by pressure from a slap with an open hand or from blast injury; it may occur from temporal bone fracture in a severe head injury. Welding sparks may cause burns to the tympanic membrane.

Haemotympanum

This is a bleed into the middle ear. It can accompany a temporal bone fracture but may occur without any bony injury. The eardrum is dull with often a bluish tinge and the patient will have a mild conductive deafness. Check hearing with the tuning forks (Chapter 3). Management is conservative and a haematoma will usually resolve. If very painful, an ENT surgeon may consider aspiration and drainage (myringotomy) (Fig. 33.1).

Perforated eardrum

Symptoms

- Pain, acute at time of rupture, usually transient.
- Deafness, not usually severe, conductive in type. The cochlea may be injured if the stapes is driven into the inner ear in which case there is sensorineural deafness. Check the hearing and do the tuning forks tests.

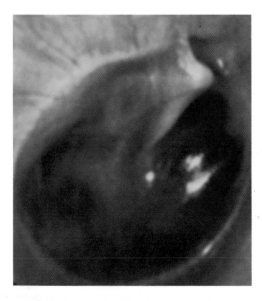

Figure 33.1 Haemotympanum.

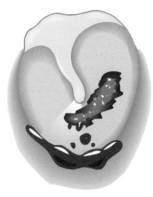

Figure 33.2 Traumatic perforation of the tympanic membrane, showing a ragged perforation with blood in the external auditory canal.

- Tinnitus may be persistent – this may be due to cochlear damage.
- Vertigo (rare).

Signs

- Bleeding from the ear.
- Blood clot in the ear canal.
- A tear in the tympanic membrane (Fig. 33.2).

Treatment of traumatic perforation: leave it alone

- Do *not* clean out the ear.
- Do *not* put in drops.
- Do *not* syringe.
- Only give antibiotics if there is evidence of infection.
- Arrange careful surveillance until the hearing has returned to normal.

Fractures of the temporal bone

Penetrating trauma may be due to gunshot wounds. Blunt trauma – road traffic accidents, falls and assault – are more common. The degree of trauma needed to fracture the temporal bone is considerable so a patient with this type of skull fracture has usually had a serious injury. Look carefully for other injuries. These fractures can be complicated by trauma to adjacent structures such as the facial nerve, the inner ear and the meninges. The patient may be unconscious. Check the facial nerve, check the hearing if you can and look for evidence of a CSF leak. As with all major trauma the priorities here are **A**irway, **B**reathing and **C**irculation before you consider definitive treatment. If you suspect a temporal bone fracture get good imaging – CT nowadays is best – and seek advice from an ENT or neurosurgeon.

> **CLINICAL PRACTICE POINTS**
>
> - Make sure a haematoma of the pinna is drained to avoid a cosmetic deformity
> - Most traumatic perforations of the eardrum heal with no long-term adverse effects
> - Temporal bone fracture denotes a severe injury.

Go to **www.lecturenoteseries.com/ENT** to test yourself using the interactive MCQs.

34

Nasal emergencies

✓ Apart from **acute sinusitis** and its complications (Chapter 18) and **trauma** (Chapter 39), **nosebleeds** (epistaxis) and **foreign bodies** are the main nasal emergencies.

Epistaxis

Nosebleeds are common; they can be persistent, serious and life-threatening.

Applied basic science

One of the functions of the nose is to warm and humidify inspired air. The nasal mucosa has a very rich blood supply and undergoes constant variation in the state of engorgement of its blood vessels. Vessels from both the internal and external carotid artery contribute, i.e. the ethmoidal arteries from the internal carotid and the greater palatine, superior labial and sphenopalatine arteries from the external carotid. These vessels form a rich plexus on the anterior part of the septum – **Little's area** or **'Keisselbachs plexus'**. Nosebleeds in young patients usually settle quickly as the blood clots and the vessels go into spasm. In elderly patients the vessels are rigid and atheromatous.

Aetiology

Some common causes are given in Table 34.1. Most nosebleeds are idiopathic. Spontaneous epistaxis is common in children and young adults; it usually arises from Little's area or from a prominent vein just below. It may be precipitated by infection or minor trauma, is easy to stop, but tends to recur. Nosebleeds in the elderly are far more difficult to treat. The bleeding site is often high up in the posterior part of the nose and on the lateral nasal wall.

Diseases of the Ear, Nose and Throat Lecture Notes, Eleventh edition. Ray Clarke. © 2014 John Wiley & Sons Ltd. Published 2014 by John Wiley & Sons, Ltd.

Table 34.1 **Causes of epistaxis**	
Local causes	**General causes**
Spontaneous	Cardiovascular conditions
Trauma	Hypertension, raised venous pressure
Tumours	Coagulation or vessel defects
Hereditary telangiectasia	Haemophilia
Nasal allergy	Leukaemia
	Anticoagulant therapy
	Thrombocytopaenia
	Fevers (rare)
	Influenza

Treatment

The treatment priorities are twofold: stop the bleeding and resuscitate the patient who has had a serious bleed.

Resuscitation and first-aid treatment

- Direct digital pressure on the lower nose compresses the vessel on the septum and will arrest bleeding from Little's area. Pressure over the nasal bones is useless.
- Treating active epistaxis is a very messy business – cover up your own clothes first. Now assess the patient and consider resuscitation. Examine the nose with a good light source. Gently remove clots and stale blood with suction. Now apply direct digital pressure to the nose for 10 min. The patient should sit leaning forward and breathe through the mouth. Discourage swallowing, which may dislodge a clot.
- If bleeding persists and the site is clearly visible, e.g. Little's area, you may be able to stop it by cautery with a silver nitrate impregnated stick (Fig. 34.1). This is easier if you first put in a plug of cotton wool or ribbon gauze soaked in lidocaine

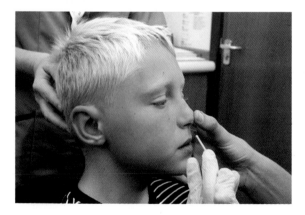

Figure 34.1 Silver nitrate stick applied to Little's area.

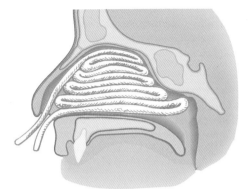

Figure 34.2 Anterior nasal packing.

and phenylephrine (Cophenalcaine TM) and leave it for 5 minutes. This also facilitates nasal packing but may not be practical if there is torrential bleeding.

Nasal packing

- If simple measures fail to control the bleeding, you will need to pack the nose. One inch ribbon gauze is traditional (Fig. 34.2). The pack is introduced along the floor of the nose and built up in loops, applying even pressure to the nasal mucosa. Alternatively, one of a variety of inflatable epistaxis 'balloons' such as the 'Brighton balloon' (Fig. 34.3) can be used. It is easier to put in but may not be as effective as a well-placed pack. Self-expanding packs (nasal tampons) such as Merocel (Fig. 34.3) which enlarge in the presence of moisture can be used.

- If bleeding continues despite adequate packing, call an ENT surgeon who may need to insert a 'post-nasal' pack. This is usually introduced under a general anaesthetic and fills the nasopharynx. A post-nasal pack is uncomfortable and causes marked airway obstruction. Patients need to be especially carefully monitored.

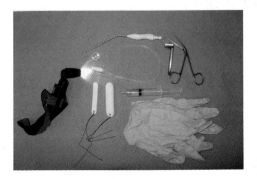

Figure 34.3 Items used to control nosebleeds.

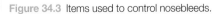

Patients with epistaxis severe enough to need packing should be admitted to hospital. With bed rest and sedation, most cases will settle. The blood pressure should be monitored and the haemoglobin level checked. Coexistent hypertension may need to be controlled.

Measures for persistent bleeding

Patients can continue to bleed despite adequate packing and resuscitation.

Surgery may be needed if the bleeding is profuse and continuous or a nasal septal deviation prevents packing. Recalcitrant bleeds may require ligation of the sphenopalatine artery by nasal endoscopic surgery. In extreme cases the ethmoidal arteries may need to be approached via the medial orbit, or the external carotid artery ligated in the neck.

Angiography and vessel embolization may rarely be considered.

Recurrent nosebleeds

Children are particularly susceptible to multiple nosebleeds. There may be minor inflammation of the nasal vestibule when daily application of a steroid/antibiotic cream or some petroleum jelly may help. Refer to an ENT surgeon for thorough nasal examination and cautery if simple measures fail.

Foreign body in the nose

Children sometimes insert foreign bodies into one or both nostrils (Fig. 34.4). The culprit may be the child, a sibling or a schoolyard or nursery chum! The objects may be hard, such as buttons, beads or ball bearings, pieces of toys, or soft – such as paper, sponge, or food particles. Organic materials soon decompose and become infected, causing symptoms more quickly.

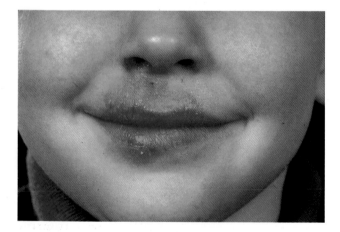

Figure 34.4 A child with a foreign body in the right nostril.

The child will often deny that he has put anything in his nose. Be suspicious!

Rarely, an adult complaining of nasal obstruction is found to have a large concretion blocking one side of the nose. This is a **rhinolith**, and consists of many layers of calcium and magnesium salts that have formed around a small central nucleus. They often contain a foreign body.

Clinical features

- Unilateral evil-smelling nasal discharge, sometimes blood-stained
- Excoriation around the nostril (vestibulitis)
- A fretful child
- Occasionally, X-ray evidence

Dangers

- Injury from clumsy attempts at removal.
- Local spread of infection – sinusitis or meningitis.
- Inhalation of foreign body – leading to lung collapse and infection. This is very rare.
- Nasal septal perforation or chemical burn of the skin around the nose– especially with leakage from 'button batteries'.

Management of suspected nasal foreign body

- Be alive to the possibility of nasal foreign bodies in small children. The child's mother may say that she suspects a foreign body. There is often uncertainty, and *When in doubt, call in expert advice.*
- If you have very good light and a cooperative child you may be able to see – and, with small nasal forceps or blunt hooks, to carefully remove – the foreign body without general anaesthetic.
- A fractious child or a child with a foreign body that has been embedded for some time will need a general anaesthetic.

CLINICAL PRACTICE POINTS

- If a mother or carer suspects a nasal foreign body, do not reassure her until you have fully inspected both nasal cavities with a good light. This may need a general anaesthetic. If in doubt, seek help.
- A button battery is potentially dangerous as corrosive fluid may leak from it. Arrange urgent removal.
- Epistaxis can kill. Particularly in elderly patients, early circulatory resuscitation, intravenous access and cross-matching may be needed before the bleed can be controlled.

 Go to **www.lecturenoteseries.com/ENT** to test yourself using the interactive MCQs.

35

Airway obstruction

The airway extends from the nasal and oral cavities to the alveoli (Fig. 35.1). Obstruction can be partial or complete. Complete airway obstruction is rapidly fatal unless dealt with very quickly. Partial airway obstruction is more common. Complete airway obstruction may be silent, and rapidly fatal, whereas partial airway obstruction is usually associated with noisy breathing – **stridor** or **stertor**.

Some of the causes of airway obstruction are shown in Figure 35.1.

Many of the clinical features of airway obstruction are nonspecific, i.e. they are not dependant on the precise aetiology. **Stridor** is a high-pitched noise caused by narrowing the larynx and upper trachea. **Stertor** is a lower pitched noise – associated with pharyngeal obstruction, and usually worse when the patient is asleep as the pharyngeal muscle tone is reduced and part of the pharynx vibrates with respiratory activity.

🔍 CLINICAL FEATURES OF AN ACUTELY OBSTRUCTED AIRWAY

- Noisy breathing (stertor or stridor).
- Confusion.
- Tachycardia.
- Increased respiratory rate (tachypnoea).
- Unconsciousness.
- Sternal recession: the sternum sinks well into the chest during inspiration, most marked in babies because of the softness of the bones in the chest wall.
- Tracheal tug: the trachea moves down in the neck during inspiration, especially in children.
- Cyanosis (a late and dangerous sign).

Diseases of the Ear, Nose and Throat Lecture Notes, Eleventh edition. Ray Clarke. © 2014 John Wiley & Sons Ltd.
Published 2014 by John Wiley & Sons, Ltd.

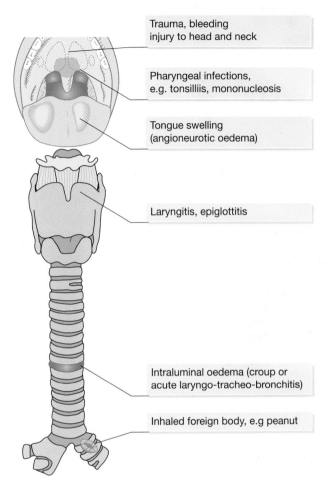

Trauma, bleeding
injury to head and neck

Pharyngeal infections,
e.g. tonsilliis, mononucleosis

Tongue swelling
(angioneurotic oedema)

Laryngitis, epiglottitis

Intraluminal oedema (croup or
acute laryngo-tracheo-bronchitis)

Inhaled foreign body, e.g peanut

Figure 35.1 Causes of airway obstruction. Source: Munir and Clarke 2013. *Ear, Nose and Throat at a Glance*. With permission of John Wiley & Sons Ltd.

Management

Relieve the obstruction

In suspected airway obstruction:

- clear the airway
- inflate the lungs
- establish an alternative airway if needed

Make sure the patient has a patent airway, either by removing the obstruction or establishing an alternative air passage (Fig. 35.2).

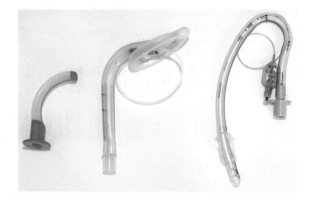

Figure 35.2 Establishing an alternative airway. A Guedel airway; a laryngeal mask; an endotracheal tube.

- **Guedel** or oral airway keeps the tongue base forward in an unconscious patient.
- An **endotracheal** airway is introduced through the mouth or the nose and guided into the trachea via the larynx. This is a skilled and often life-saving procedure (endotracheal intubation).
- **A laryngeal mask airway** is introduced through the mouth. The mask rests on the laryngeal inlet permitting ventilation.
- An emergency tracheotomy is nowadays very rarely needed, but in an extreme emergency it may be possible to perforate the membrane between the thyroid cartilage and the cricoid cartilage (**cricothyroidotomy**; Fig. 30.2 Chapter 30).

Measures that may help support the patient until the obstruction is overcome

- **Oxygen therapy**: will not overcome obstruction but can prevent hypoxia in the short term.
- **Adrenaline**: nebulized adrenaline can help to open the small airways in particular.
- **Steroids**: oral prednisolone or dexamethasone can reduce airway mucosal oedema.

> **CLINICAL PRACTICE POINT**
>
> - The most important measure in managing acute airway obstruction is to remove the obstruction. If you cannot do this, try to establish an alternative airway until the patient can have definitive treatment.

 Go to **www.lecturenoteseries.com/ENT** to test yourself using the interactive MCQs.

36

Airway obstruction in infants and children

✓ Upper airway obstruction (see Box 36.1) in children is dangerous and may progress rapidly. Make a firm diagnosis and take the appropriate action without delay.

Causes of upper airway obstruction in infancy

Supralaryngeal causes

Choanal atresia

Failure of posterior canalization of the nasal airways results in severe neonatal airway obstruction relieved by crying. This condition is fortunately rare –1 in 8000 live births. Surgical correction will be needed to enable the baby to feed. (Figs 36.1 and 36.2)

Micrognathia

Underdevelopment of the mandible as in Pierre Robin sequence (which includes cleft palate) or Treacher–Collins syndrome (see Chapter 5) results in posterior displacement of the tongue (glossoptosis) and oropharyngeal obstruction. The neonate may asphyxiate unless corrective measures – e.g. insertion of an oral airway or a nasopharyngeal tube – are taken.

Adeno-tonsillar hypertrophy

Large tonsils and adenoids may occlude the naso-oropharyngeal airway to a serious degree. This may result in obstructive apnoea during sleep, with loud snoring punctuated by periods of silence followed by a large gasp – Chapter 24.

Diseases of the Ear, Nose and Throat Lecture Notes, Eleventh edition. Ray Clarke. © 2014 John Wiley & Sons Ltd.
Published 2014 by John Wiley & Sons, Ltd.

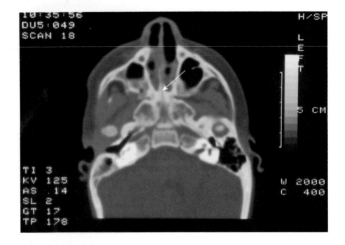

Figure 36.1 CT scan of bilateral choanal atresia.

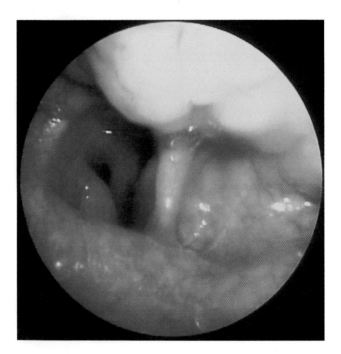

Figure 36.2 Endoscopic view of unilateral congenital posterior choanal atresia. The atretic plate can be clearly seen, and on the patent side the posterior ends of the inferior and middle turbinates are visible.

Box 36.1 **Signs of airway obstruction**

- **Stertor** produced by obstruction in the throat, i.e. above the larynx, is a low-pitched choking type of noise.

- **Stridor** is a high-pitched sound produced by narrowing within the more rigid confines of the larynx or trachea. In laryngeal obstruction the stridor is inspiratory; in tracheal lesions it is usually both inspiratory and expiratory.

- Use of **accessory muscles of respiration**.

- Intercostal and sternal **recession** (Fig. 36.3). The sternum may be sucked in almost to the vertebrae in the child's attempts to breathe.

- **Pallor**, sweating and restlessness.

- **Tachycardia**.

- **Cyanosis**. Examine the child in adequate lighting, preferably daylight. The lips particularly will show the dusky colouration, which may be very subtle. Cyanosis is a late and dangerous sign. Don't wait for it.

- **Exhaustion** – a late stage in asphyxia, which should be avoided. The child makes less effort to breathe, stridor and recession becomes less pronounced and apnoea is not far off.

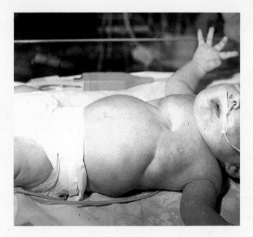

Figure 36.3 Baby with severe upper airway obstruction. Note the sternal recession and paradoxical abdominal movement.

Laryngo-tracheal causes

Congenital

- **Laryngomalacia** (floppy larynx, Fig. 36.4): The stridor starts at or shortly after birth and is due to inward collapse of the soft laryngeal tissues on inspiration. It usually resolves by the age of 2 years, but meanwhile the baby may have respiratory

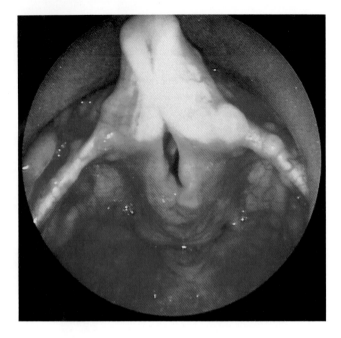

Figure 36.4 Laryngomalacia. Note the insuction of the supraglottic structures, causing airway narrowing.

difficulties. Diagnosis is confirmed by laryngoscopy without intubation when the supraglottic collapse is seen on inspiration. It can be relieved by division or excision of the membrane between the epiglottis and the arytenoids (aryepiglottic folds).

- **Congenital subglottic stenosis**: This occurs at the level of the cricoid cartilage. There will be stridor from birth and the stenosis may be visible on a lateral X-ray of the neck. Diagnosis is confirmed by laryngoscopy.
- **Laryngeal webs/cysts:** Laryngeal webs are usually anteriorly situated (Fig. 36.5) and if large can cause severe stridor and obstruction. The most extreme degree of webbing, atresia, is fatal without a tracheotomy. Laryngeal cysts may be congenital or the result of endotracheal intubation.
- **Tracheal Compression**: A vascular ring – or a mediastinal mass- may constrict the trachea.
- **Tracheomalacia**: The tracheal cartilage may be unduly soft and close off during respiration-particularly in premature babies.

Acquired

- **Foreign body** (Figs 36.6 and 36.7): Always suspect the sudden onset of stridor in a previously healthy child as due to a foreign body until proved otherwise. A history of choking and coughing, especially while eating, should alert you to the

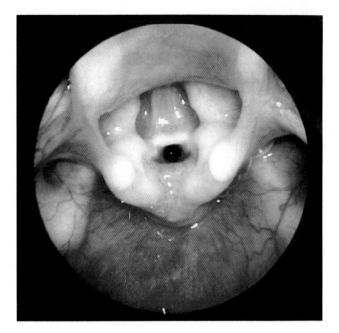

Figure 36.5 Anterior laryngeal web.

likelihood of aspiration; peanuts are particularly dangerous and should *never* be given to youngsters. A foreign body in the bronchus may permit some air entry but obstruct it mainly in expiration. This can cause a 'ball valve' effect with hyperinflation of one lung on chest X-ray – the so-called 'obstructive emphysema' (Fig. 36.7). Examination and chest X-rays may be entirely normal and the only way to exclude a foreign body in the bronchus is by bronchoscopy. A larger foreign body may lodge in the larynx and cause severe respiratory distress. It may be possible to get the child to expel it by the Heimlich manoeuvre (compression of the upper abdomen to raise intrathoracic pressure) but if this fails, emergency endoscopy or tracheotomy will be necessary.

- **Acute laryngitis, acute epiglottitis and laryngotracheobronchitis**: Described in Chapter 26.
- **Subglottic stenosis** (Fig. 36.8): Subglottic stenosis is now seen most commonly in low-birth-weight babies who have had prolonged ventilation by endotracheal tube. Treatment is highly specialized and entails some form of laryngotracheal surgery to reconstruct the airway.

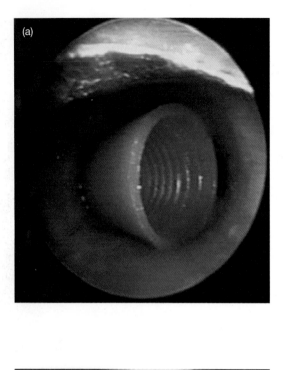

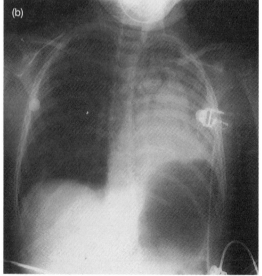

Figure 36.6 (a) Part of a ball-point pen lodged in the left main bronchus as seen at bronchoscopy. (b) The chest film shows loss of lung volume and mediastinal shift.

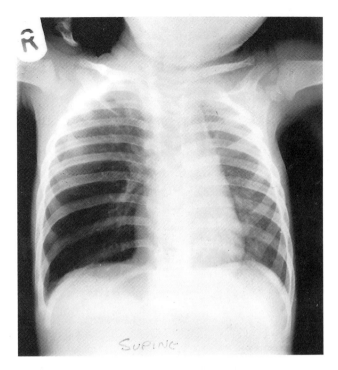

Figure 36.7 Foreign body in the right main bronchus in a baby of 6 months. Note that the right lung is hyperinflated and therefore darker on the X-ray.

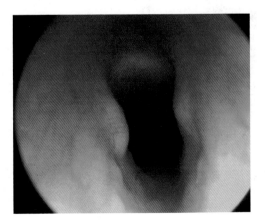

Figure 36.8 Endoscopic view showing moderate subglottic stenosis and small ductal cysts following ventilation as a neonate.

- **Recurrent respiratory papillomatosis** (Fig. 36.9): This is a serious condition caused by the human papilloma virus (HPV) types 6 and 11. The virus is transmitted through the mother's birth canal. Suspect papillomatosis in a child with progressive hoarseness or aphonia and airway obstruction. There may be little stridor since the mass of papillomas is too soft to vibrate the air column. Removal of the papillomas is best accomplished using a microdebrider at laryngotracheoscopy. The papillomas have a strong tendency to recur. As girls in most Western countries are now vaccinated against HPV this condition may become even more rare.

Management of airway obstruction

The management of airway insufficiency depends on the severity. Severe obstruction needs immediate airway support by oxygen, endotracheal intubation or very rarely tracheotomy – Chapter 35.

Neonates may be intubated without the need for general anaesthesia but great care must be taken not to damage the larynx and cause further obstruction from haematoma or oedema. Older children, unless so anoxic as to be unconscious, will require general anaesthesia for intubation, and at the same time the larynx, trachea and bronchi should be inspected. Inspection of the airways in cases of respiratory obstruction calls for the highest degree of co-operation between surgeon and anaesthetist. The larynx is inspected using a rigid paediatric laryngoscope and Hopkins rod telescope (Fig. 36.10). Bronchoscopy in babies and children has been facilitated greatly by the introduction of ventilating bronchoscopes, which allow coupling to an anaesthetic circuit (Fig. 36.11).

The diagnosis is then usually apparent and further management can be directed appropriately.

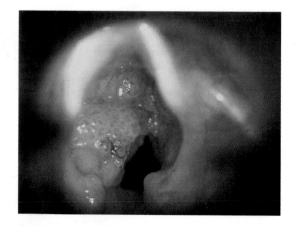

Figure 36.9 A large mass of papillomata on the left vocal cord.

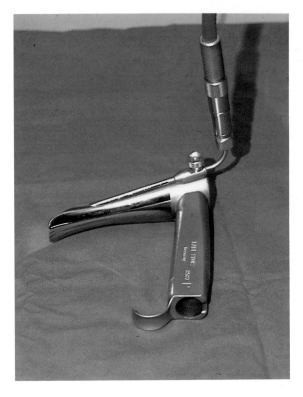

Figure 36.10 A small laryngoscope used for examining young children.

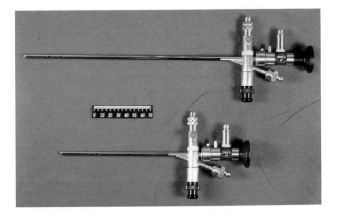

Figure 36.11 Ventilating bronchoscopes. Note the telescope, the side channel for instrumentation and the inlet for anaesthetic gases and oxygen.

CLINICAL PRACTICE POINTS

- Any child with stridor is potentially at risk. Determine the cause. Not all children 'grow out' of a tendency to stridor.
- Beware the exhausted child whose stridor has quietened. He may be near asphyxiation.
- Never allow young children near peanuts or other small objects they may inhale and advise parents and carers accordingly. An inhaled foreign body can be fatal.
- Bilateral choanal atresia is a life-threatening emergency. Secure an oral airway and refer to ENT immediately.

 Go to **www.lecturenoteseries.com/ENT** to test yourself using the interactive MCQs.

37

Pharyngeal and oesophageal ingested foreign bodies

Children – and occasionally adults – may ingest coins, toys or more bizarre objects (Fig. 37.1). If inhaled they may be expelled by coughing. More seriously they may cause airway obstruction or impact in a bronchus (see Chapter 36). Some will impact in the pharynx or oesophagus. Small bones – especially fishbones and small particles of chicken bone – can get stuck in the pharynx, notably the tongue base and the tonsil. They may scratch or tear the pharyngeal mucosa before passing down into the stomach. They can also lodge in the pharynx or oesophagus, where they may lead to perforation, mediastinitis or abscess, or even fatal penetration of the aorta.

Elderly patients may swallow their dentures. Sometimes poorly chewed food – especially a bolus of meat – can obstruct the oesophagus. Fish, poultry and other bones are often inadvertently swallowed. An impacted foreign body in the pharynx or oesophagus is potentially very serious.

Clinical features

- May be a clear history, but not always.
- Feeling of a 'scratch' or sharp 'point' on swallowing – especially with fish or chicken bone.
- Painful swallow – odynophagia.
- Dysphagia – incomplete or complete, i.e. patient may be drooling and unable to swallow saliva.
- Rarely a bolus stuck at the entrance to the oesophagus can cause pressure on the trachea and airway obstruction.

Diseases of the Ear, Nose and Throat Lecture Notes, Eleventh edition. Ray Clarke. © 2014 John Wiley & Sons Ltd.
Published 2014 by John Wiley & Sons, Ltd.

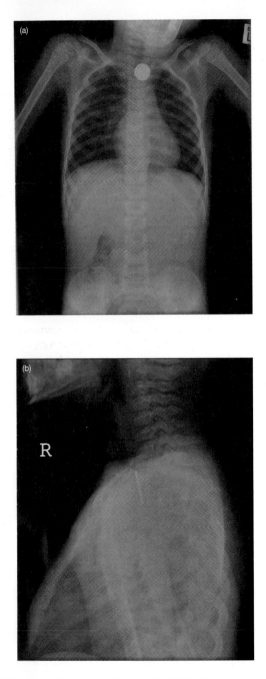

Figure 37.1 Coin in the oesophagus. AP (a) and lateral (b) view.

Management

Sharp foreign body

If a patient presents with a history of having swallowed a sharp foreign body – e.g. a bone – he will complain of soreness in the throat. It may be very difficult to decide whether a foreign body has simply caused an abrasion and has passed on, or is impacted.

Take a careful history, noting the nature of the suspected foreign body (is it radio-opaque?) and the time of ingestion.

Examine the pharynx and larynx. Pay particular attention to the tonsils and tongue base. (Fish bones often stick here.) A foreign body lodged in the cervical oesophagus will cause pain on gently pressing the larynx against the spine.

X-ray the chest and neck (lateral view) – remember that plastic and some fish bones will not show.

If there is any doubt, seek expert advice.

Indications for pharyngo-oesophagoscopy

- Dysphagia.
- Suspected foreign body on X-ray.
- Persistent symptoms.

Impacted food bolus

Dysphagia and drooling suggest complete oesophageal obstruction. A carbonated drink may help, as may a gentle sedative such as diazepam (by injection). If the bolus has impacted and won't move, arrange admission to hospital for endoscopic removal.

Q CLINICAL PRACTICE POINT

- Carefully inspect the tongue base and the tonsil in a patient with a feeling of a small bone 'stuck in the throat'. You may be able to see it with a good light and remove it with a forceps.

Go to **www.lecturenoteseries.com/ENT** to test yourself using the interactive MCQs.

38

Neck trauma

Types of trauma

- **Penetrating** neck injuries due to gunshot wounds and stabbing are now all too common. Penetrating injuries may result in damage to nerves (e.g. the facial nerve), vessels, ducts (the parotid duct) and the midline viscuses (larynx, trachea, pharynx and oesophagus). Each may need surgical attention by wound exploration but the main priorities in the early management of patients with neck trauma are identification and resuscitation.
- **Blunt trauma** can be due to road traffic accidents, strangulation or contact sports injuries. (Fig. 38.1)
- **Iatrogenic laryngotracheal injuries:** Long-term endotracheal intubation of patients on intensive care units can cause ischaemia and scarring of the laryngotracheal mucosa. This can reduce and permanently scar the airway, especially in children where the tracheal lumen is in any case narrow. Prolonged endotracheal ventilation for broncho-pulmonary dysplasia and respiratory distress syndrome has inevitably resulted in cases of laryngeal stenosis in tiny infants, especially premature babies. More recently, the avoidance of irritant tubes, awareness of the need to control cuff pressures and a tendency to use smaller calibre endotracheal tubes have led to a reduction in the incidence of airway stenosis. Tracheotomy can be complicated by long-term laryngo-tracheal stenosis.
- Other causes of traumatic damage to the neck structures are **inhaled flames** or **hot vapours** and **swallowed corrosives**.

Diagnosis

Laryngotracheal trauma is often missed amid other serious injuries. Consider it when the neck is injured. Fractures of the larynx will produce hoarseness and stridor, and urgent tracheotomy may be needed. In cases of cut throat, it may be possible to intubate the larynx through the wound, prior to formal tracheotomy and

Diseases of the Ear, Nose and Throat Lecture Notes, Eleventh edition. Ray Clarke. © 2014 John Wiley & Sons Ltd.
Published 2014 by John Wiley & Sons, Ltd.

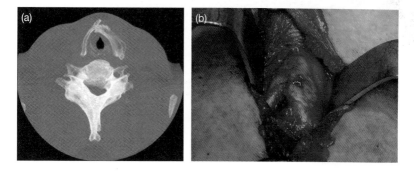

Figure 38.1 CT scan and operation showing fracture of the thyroid cartilage and the result of repair by wiring. A rugby injury.

laryngeal repair (Fig. 38.2). Occasionally a penetrating injury can sever the trachea but not be immediately recognized as the two sections are still apposed.

Management

- **ABC** – **A**irway, **B**reathing, **C**irculation.
- The airway can be at risk and there can be profuse bleeding from a severed vessel. These need to be attended to before any other measures are considered.
- Establish an airway by intubation or tracheostomy.
- Laryngeal repair may be needed later.

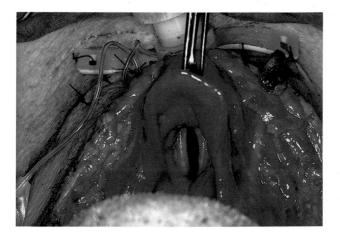

Figure 38.2 A self-inflicted cut throat, giving a good view of the anatomy.

CLINICAL PRACTICE POINT

- Always look for signs of laryngotracheal trauma in a patient with neck injuries.

 Go to **www.lecturenoteseries.com/ENT** to test yourself using the interactive MCQs.

39

Maxillofacial trauma

Facial injuries are common. Blunt facial trauma due to assault, sporting injuries, and road traffic accidents are common. The nasal bones fracture easily but more severe trauma can cause maxillary and mandibular fractures.

Features of nasal injury

- Bleeding
- Injury to the nasal septum
- Fractures of the nasal bones

Fracture of the nasal bones (Fig. 39.1)

The fracture is often simple but can be comminuted with multiple fragments. There may be an open wound in the skin over the nasal bones – compound fracture.

Clinical features

- Bruising of the skin and subcutaneous tissues over the nasal bones.
- Tenderness over the fracture site.
- Mobility of the nose.
- Deformity, i.e. the shape of the nose has altered (not always present).

Diseases of the Ear, Nose and Throat Lecture Notes, Eleventh edition. Ray Clarke. © 2014 John Wiley & Sons Ltd. Published 2014 by John Wiley & Sons, Ltd.

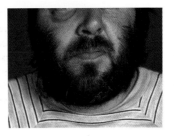

Figure 39.1 Patient with nasal fracture showing gross displacement of the nasal bones to the left and bruising below the right eye.

Treatment of nasal fracture

Early treatment

The patient may have had multiple injuries and need resuscitation. Fractured noses usually bleed. Control this first. Examine carefully to make sure there are no other facial fractures, e.g. orbital rim, mandible. Clean lacerations meticulously to avoid tattooing with dirt and carefully repair them.

Manipulation of fracture

Dislocation of the nasal bone is common. If a previously straight nose is bent following an injury, it must be broken. If it is not bent after an injury, the bones will heal and there will be no external deformity. Stand behind and above the patient's head and look down on the nose. If there is no deformity, no manipulation or splinting is needed. If the nasal bones are displaced, plan a reduction of the fracture. Nasal injury often results in deviation of the nasal septum, causing airway obstruction. This rarely needs immediate treatment. If there is no external deformity an ENT surgeon will arrange septal surgery – 'septoplasty' – after a period of weeks or months. If there is a complex injury to both the bones and the cartilage a good result may only be obtained by simultaneous correction of both – before the bones have set. Nasal fractures can be reduced immediately after the injury by simple manipulation, but the appropriate medical attendant is rarely present. More often, the patient presents himself some time later, by which time oedema may obscure the extent of any deformity and pain precludes manipulation. Oedema will settle over 5–7 days. Make sure the patient sees an ENT surgeon within a week of injury. After 2 weeks, the bone may be fixed and deformity may be permanent. The optimum timing for straightening the nose is usually 7–10 days after the injury. This can be done under local anaesthesia but general anaesthesia is usually employed. Depressed nasal fractures will require elevation with forceps. External splinting is rarely needed.

Septal haematoma

Sometimes, soon after a punch on the nose, the victim complains of very severe nasal obstruction. This may be caused by a septal haematoma – the result of bleeding between the two layers of muco-perichondrium covering the septum. It is often (but not always) associated with a fracture of the septum. The appearance is quite distinctive. Both nasal passages are obliterated by a boggy, pink or dull red swelling replacing the septum. Treatment may not be needed for a very small haematoma, but a large one requires incision along the base of the septum, evacuation of the clot, insertion of a drain and nasal packing to approximate the septal coverings of muco-perichondrium. Antibiotic cover should be considered to avert the development of a septal abscess. At worst this will cause 'saddling' of the nose as the cartilage necroses. The patient should be warned that there may be permanent deformity of the nose.

Late treatment of nasal fractures

If a patient with a fractured nose presents months or years after injury, manipulation is clearly not possible, and formal corrective surgery to both the bones and the cartilage – septorhinoplasty – (SRP, Chapter 21) is the only way to correct the deformity. It is a difficult procedure and it is far better to treat a nasal fracture well at the time of injury.

Injuries of the maxilla

LeFort fractures

A good deal more trauma is needed to cause a maxillary fracture. The bones tend to follow one of three patterns, hence these fractures are classified as LeFort type 1, 2 and 3 (Figs. 39.2, 39.3 and 39.4). The patient will usually have a history of

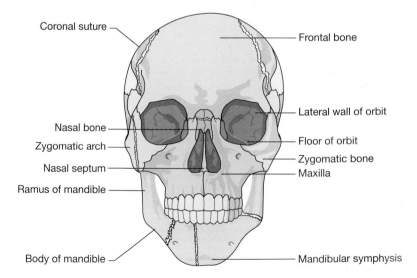

Figure 39.2 The facial skeleton, showing common fracture sites in the zygoma and the mandible.

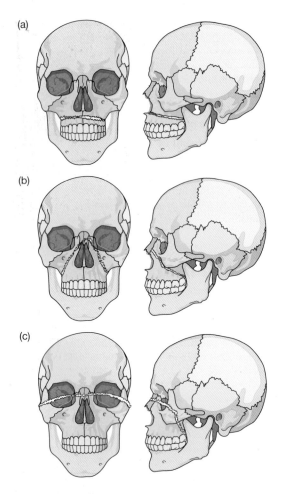

Figure 39.3 Common facial fractures: (a) LeFort type 1, also known as 'floating palate' fracture; (b) LeFort type 2, a severe injury usually involving the orbital rim; and (c) LeFort type 3, also known as craniofacial dysfunction, a very severe injury.

severe trauma; there may be epistaxis, extensive facial bruising, and malloclusion when he attempts to close his mouth. Le-Fort11 and 111 fractures especially may be associated with head injury, cerebrospinal fluid leaks, airway obstruction and eye complications.

Zygomatic bone or 'malar' fracture

This is a fracture of the zygoma, the bone that forms the malar eminence of the face. It often results from a blow from an assailant's fist.

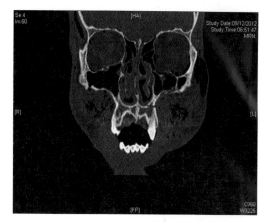

Figure 39.4 A Le Fort 1 fracture with some comminution and surgical emphysema.

Orbital 'blow-out' fracture (Fig. 39.5)

Caused by a blunt force such as a squash or tennis ball, a fist, a hockey stick or a cork, the intra-orbital pressure suddenly increases and the thin bones break causing the contents of the globe – especially the orbital muscles – to herniate downwards or laterally, sometimes trapping the contents. The patient may complain of diplopia and there may be a palpable deformity or a visible asymmetery of the eyes. Be vigilant as these injuries can be missed. Good quality imaging is important in the management of maxilla-mandibular fractures, in contrast with nasal fractures where imaging is of limited value.

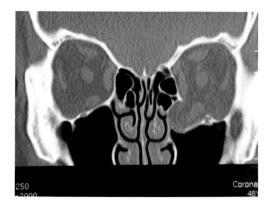

Figure 39.5 'Blowout' fracture of the orbit. Note the defect in the floor of the orbit. The contents of the orbit have herniated into the maxillary sinus. This fracture needs skilled emergency management to preserve vision.

Fractures of the mandible (Figs 39.6 and 39.7)

These are usually the result of severe trauma, e.g. assault or road traffic accidents. The patient will complain of pain. There may be malocclusion of the teeth and mucosal tears of the mouth. Mandibular fractures may be one of a number of injuries in multiple trauma.

Management of maxilla-mandibular fractures

- Recognition and resuscitation are the priorities.
- Remember the ABC of trauma care. Establish a good **A**irway and ensure **B**reathing and **C**irculation are adequate.
- Definitive treatment is largely the preserve of specialist maxillofacial surgeons.
- Open Reduction and Internal Fixation (ORIF) are often needed

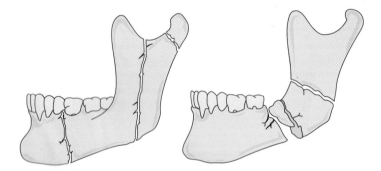

Figure 39.6 Mandibular fractures.

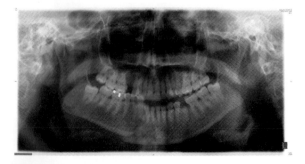

Figure 39.7 Mandibular fracture.

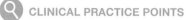

CLINICAL PRACTICE POINTS

- Check a patient with a nasal injury for other facial fractures.
- Look for a septal haematoma and if you suspect one refer immediately to ENT.
- Make sure nasal fractures are seen by an ENT surgeon within 7 days of the injury.
- X-rays are of doubtful value in simple nasal fractures. Decide whether the patient needs a reduction based on whether or not there is a visible external deformity.
- A patient with a maxillary or mandibular fracture has had severe trauma

Go to www.lecturenoteseries.com/ENT to test yourself using the interactive MCQs.

Index

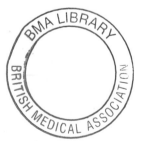